Imaging of Incidentalomas

Guest Editor

ALEC J. MEGIBOW, MD, MPH, FACR

RADIOLOGIC CLINICS OF NORTH AMERICA

www.radiologic.theclinics.com

Consulting Editor
FRANK H. MILLER, MD

March 2011 • Volume 49 • Number 2

SAUNDERS an imprint of ELSEVIER, Inc.

W.B. SAUNDERS COMPANY
A Division of Elsevier Inc.

1600 John F. Kennedy Boulevard • Suite 1800 • Philadelphia, Pennsylvania 19103-2899

http://www.theclinics.com

RADIOLOGIC CLINICS OF NORTH AMERICA Volume 49, Number 2
March 2011 ISSN 0033-8389, ISBN 13: 978-1-4557-0501-6

Editor: Barton Dudlick
Developmental Editor: Donald E. Mumford

Radiologic Clinics of North America (ISSN 0033-8389) is published bimonthly by Elsevier Inc., 360 Park Avenue South, New York, NY 10010-1710. Months of issue are January, March, May, July, September, and November. Periodicals postage paid at New York, NY and additional mailing offices. Subscription prices are USD 386 per year for US individuals, USD 610 per year for US institutions, USD 185 per year for US students and residents, USD 450 per year for Canadian individuals, USD 766 per year for Canadian institutions, USD 556 per year for international individuals, USD 766 per year for international institutions, and USD 266 per year for Canadian and foreign students/residents. To receive student and resident rate, orders must be accompanied by name of affiliated institution, date of term and the signature of program/residency coordinatior on institution letterhead. Orders will be billed at individual rate until proof of status is received. Foreign air speed delivery is included in all *Clinics* subscription prices. All prices are subject to change without notice. **POSTMASTER:** Send address changes to *Radiologic Clinics of North America*, Elsevier Health Sciences Division, Subscription Customer Service, 3251 Riverport Lane, Maryland Heights, MO63043. **Customer Service: Telephone: 1-800-654-2452** (U.S. and Canada); **1-314-447-8871** (outside U.S. and Canada). **Fax: 1-314-447-8029. E-mail: journalscustomerservice-usa@ elsevier.com** (for print support); **journalsonlinesupport-usa@elsevier.com** (for online support).

Reprints. For copies of 100 or more of articles in this publication, please contact the Commercial Reprints Department, Elsevier Inc., 360 Park Avenue South, New York, New York 10010-1710. Tel.: (+1) 212-633-3812; Fax: (+1) 212-462-1935; E-mail: reprints@elsevier.com.

Radiologic Clinics of North America also published in Greek Paschalidis Medical Publications, Athens, Greece.

Radiologic Clinics of North America is covered in *MEDLINE/PubMed (Index Medicus), EMBASE/Excerpta Medica, Current Contents/Life Sciences, Current Contents/Clinical Medicine, RSNA Index to Imaging Literature, BIOSIS, Science Citation Index,* and *ISI/BIOMED.*

Printed and bound by CPI Group (UK) Ltd, Croydon, CR0 4YY

Transferred to Digital Print 2011

Contributors

CONSULTING EDITOR

FRANK H. MILLER, MD
Professor of Radiology; Chief, Body Imaging
Section and Fellowship Program and GI
Radiology, Medical Director MRI, Department
of Radiology, Northwestern University Feinberg
School of Medicine, Chicago, Illinois

GUEST EDITOR

ALEC J. MEGIBOW, MD, MPH, FACR
Professor of Radiology and Director, Outpatient
Imaging Services, Department of Radiology,
New York University Langone Medical Center,
New York, New York

AUTHORS

SAMEER AHMED
Johns Hopkins School of Medicine, Baltimore,
Maryland

JEFFREY B. ALPERT, MD
Fellow, Thoracic Imaging Section, Department
of Radiology, New York University Langone
Medical Center, New York, New York

MARK E. BAKER, MD
Department of Radiology, Cleveland Clinic
Foundation, Cleveland, Ohio

LINCOLN L. BERLAND, MD, FACR
Professor Emeritus and Vice-Chairman for
Quality Improvement and Patient Safety,
Department of Radiology; Chief, University
of Alabama at Birmingham, Birmingham,
Alabama

JONATHAN W. BERLIN, MD
Department of Radiology, North Shore
University Health System; Associate
Professor of Radiology, Pritzker School
of Medicine, University of Chicago,
Evanston, Illinois

LEONARD BERLIN, MD, FACR
Professor of Radiology, Department of Radiology,
Rush Medical College, Chicago; Vice-Chair,
Department of Radiology, NorthShore University
HealthSystem, Skokie Hospital, Skokie, Illinois

ALEXANDER DING, MD, MS
Radiology Resident, Department of Radiology,
Massachusetts General Hospital, Boston,
Massachusetts

JONATHAN D. EISENBERG, BA
Research Associate, Department of Radiology,
Institute for Technology Assessment,
Massachusetts General Hospital, Boston,
Massachusetts

ELLIOT K. FISHMAN, MD
Russell H. Morgan Department of Radiology
and Radiological Science, Johns Hopkins
Hospital, Baltimore, Maryland

RICHARD M. GORE, MD
Department of Radiology, North Shore University
Health System; Professor of Radiology, Pritzker
School of Medicine, University of Chicago,
Evanston, Illinois

KAREN M. HORTON, MD
Russell H. Morgan Department of Radiology
and Radiological Science, Johns Hopkins
Hospital, Baltimore, Maryland

GARY M. ISRAEL, MD
Professor, Department of Radiology, Yale
University School of Medicine; Chief of CT,
New Haven, Connecticut

WILLIAM W. MAYO-SMITH, MD
Professor of Diagnostic Imaging, Department
of Diagnostic Imaging, Rhode Island Hospital —
Warren Alpert Medical School of Brown
University, Providence, Rhode Island

ALEC J. MEGIBOW, MD, MPH, FACR
Professor of Radiology and Director, Outpatient
Imaging Services, Department of Radiology,
New York University Langone Medical Center,
New York, New York

UDAY K. MEHTA, MD
Department of Radiology, North Shore
University Health System; Associate
Professor of Radiology, Pritzker School
of Medicine, University of Chicago,
Evanston, Illinois

DAVID P. NAIDICH, MD
Professor of Radiology and Medicine,
Thoracic Imaging Section, Department
of Radiology, New York University Langone
Medical Center, New York, New York

GERALDINE M. NEWMARK, MD
Department of Radiology, North Shore University
Health System; Associate Professor of Radiology,
Pritzker School of Medicine, University of Chicago,
Evanston, Illinois

PARI V. PANDHARIPANDE, MD, MPH
Assistant Professor of Radiology, Harvard Medical
School; Department of Radiology, Institute for
Technology Assessment, Massachusetts General
Hospital, Boston, Massachusetts

STUART G. SILVERMAN, MD
Professor of Radiology, Harvard Medical School;
Director, Abdominal Imaging and Intervention;
Director, CT Scan, Department of Radiology,
Brigham and Women's Hospital, Boston,
Massachusetts

JULIE H. SONG, MD
Associate Professor of Diagnostic Imaging
(Clinical), Department of Diagnostic Imaging,
Rhode Island Hospital — Warren Alpert Medical
School of Brown University, Providence, Rhode
Island

ANDREW TAYLOR, MD
Department of Radiology, Virginia Commonwealth
University Medical Center, Richmond, Virginia

KIRAN H. THAKRAR, MD
Department of Radiology, North Shore University
Health System; Assistant Professor of Radiology,
Pritzker School of Medicine, University of Chicago,
Evanston, Illinois

Contents

There has been a dramatically increased awareness of the substantial clinical challenges posed by incidental findings found on cross-sectional imaging. In 2006, an
Incidental Findings Committee was organized under the Body Imaging Commission
in the American College of Radiology to create a consistent and rational approach to
these findings. This article describes the formation, process of developing recommendations, and future tasks of this committee.

With the advent of high-resolution computed tomography, magnetic resonance
imaging, and ultrasonography, the frequency of radiologists' serendipitous discovery of incidentalomas is increasing. If the radiologist believes an incidentaloma is
of no clinical significance, then making mention of it in the radiological report may
possibly lead to a cascade of tests, biopsies, and other surgical procedures, which
occasionally can cause serious complications. But if the incidentaloma is not reported and it later turns out to be an early carcinoma or sign of other significant
disease, the patient's health may be irreversibly jeopardized. In either case, medical
malpractice litigation could well ensue.

Practitioners in all medical disciplines recognize the high frequency of incidentally
detected findings. Although some findings are discovered on physical examination,
an increasing majority are detected at imaging performed for another indication.
With increasing federal scrutiny on the net value of imaging services, the costs
and benefits of incidental findings need to be more rigorously quantified. In this article, the authors examine current related work on imaging expenditures for incidental findings and provide a framework for future investigations that will efficiently and
substantially advance the knowledge in this field.

With continued improvement of high-resolution multidetector computed tomography imaging, there is an increasing number of unsuspected thoracic findings.
Although many of these findings are of little clinical significance, other findings
such as small incidental lung nodules require additional imaging to exclude more
worrisome causes, often resulting in greater exposure to ionizing radiation, increased cost, and patient anxiety. Although greater uniformity among radiologists

regarding likely benign findings may help reduce unnecessary imaging studies, the lack of clear follow-up guidelines for many findings suggests that further investigation is needed in some areas.

Incidental renal masses are extremely common. Although most represent benign renal cysts, not all incidental renal masses are benign. Most renal cell carcinomas are discovered incidentally when an imaging examination is performed to evaluate a nonrenal complaint. Therefore, differentiating incidental benign renal masses from those that are potentially malignant is important. There are well-established, time-tested, image-based criteria that can be used to diagnose most renal masses definitively. However, some renal masses remain indeterminate even after a thorough evaluation with imaging. This article discusses the evaluation, diagnosis, and treatment options of the incidental renal mass.

GOAL STATEMENT

The goal of the *Radiologic Clinics of North America* is to keep practicing radiologists and radiology residents up to date with current clinical practice in radiology by providing timely articles reviewing the state of the art in patient care.

ACCREDITATION

The *Radiologic Clinics of North America* is planned and implemented in accordance with the Essential Areas and Policies of the Accreditation Council for Continuing Medical Education (ACCME) through the joint sponsorship of the University of Virginia School of Medicine and Elsevier. The University of Virginia School of Medicine is accredited by the ACCME to provide continuing medical education for physicians.

The University of Virginia School of Medicine designates this educational activity for a maximum of 15 *AMA PRA Category 1 Credits*™ for each issue, 90 credits per year. Physicians should only claim credit commensurate with the extent of their participation in the activity.

The American Medical Association has determined that physicians not licensed in the US who participate in this CME activity are eligible for a maximum of *15 AMA PRA Category 1 Credits*™ for each issue, 90 credits per year.

Credit can be earned by reading the text material, taking the CME examination online at http://www.theclinics.com/home/cme, and completing the evaluation. After taking the test, you will be required to review any and all incorrect answers. Following completion of the test and evaluation, your credit will be awarded and you may print your certificate.

FACULTY DISCLOSURE/CONFLICT OF INTEREST

The University of Virginia School of Medicine, as an ACCME accredited provider, endorses and strives to comply with the Accreditation Council for Continuing Medical Education (ACCME) Standards of Commercial Support, Commonwealth of Virginia statutes, University of Virginia policies and procedures, and associated federal and private regulations and guidelines on the need for disclosure and monitoring of proprietary and financial interests that may affect the scientific integrity and balance of content delivered in continuing medical education activities under our auspices.

The University of Virginia School of Medicine requires that all CME activities accredited through this institution be developed independently and be scientifically rigorous, balanced and objective in the presentation/discussion of its content, theories and practices.

All authors/editors participating in an accredited CME activity are expected to disclose to the readers relevant financial relationships with commercial entities occurring within the past 12 months (such as grants or research support, employee, consultant, stock holder, member of speakers bureau, etc.). The University of Virginia School of Medicine will employ appropriate mechanisms to resolve potential conflicts of interest to maintain the standards of fair and balanced education to the reader. Questions about specific strategies can be directed to the Office of Continuing Medical Education, University of Virginia School of Medicine, Charlottesville, Virginia.

The faculty and staff of the University of Virginia Office of Continuing Medical Education have no financial affiliations to disclose.

The authors/editors listed below have identified no financial or professional relationships for themselves or their spouse/partner:

Sameer Ahmed; Jeffrey B. Alpert, MD; Leonard Berlin, MD; Alexander Ding, MD, MS; Barton Dudlick, (Acquisitions Editor); Jonathan D. Eisenberg, BA; Richard M. Gore, MD; Karen M. Horton, MD; Gary M. Israel, MD; William W. Mayo-Smith, MD; Uday K. Mehta, MD; Frank H. Miller, MD (Consulting Editor); David P. Naidich, MD; Geraldine M. Newmark, MD; Pari V. Pandharipande, MD, MPH; Stuart G. Silverman, MD; Julie H. Song, MD; Andrew Taylor, MD; and Kiran H. Thakrar, MD.

The authors/editors listed below have identified the following financial or professional relationships for themselves or their spouse/partner:

Mark E. Baker, MD is on the Advisory Committee/Board for Bracco, and is an industry funded research/investigator for Siemens Medical Systems.
Lincoln L. Berland, MD is a consultant and is on the Advisory Committee/Board for Nuance, Inc.
Jonathan W. Berlin, MD is on the Advisory Board and is a stockholder for Nuance Communications.
Elliot K. Fishman, MD is an industry funded research/investigator for Siemens Medical Solutions and GE.
Klaus D. Hagspiel, MD (Test Author) is an industry funded reseach/investigator for Siemens Medical Solutions.
Alec J. Megibow, MD, MPH (Guest Editor) is a consultant for Bracco Diagnostics, and is on the Advisory Board/Committee for Siemens Medical Solutions.

Disclosure of Discussion of Non-FDA Approved Uses for Pharmaceutical Products and/or Medical Devices.
The University of Virginia School of Medicine, as an ACCME provider, requires that all faculty presenters identify and disclose any off-label uses for pharmaceutical and medical device products. The University of Virginia School of Medicine recommends that each physician fully review all the available data on new products or procedures prior to clinical use.

TO ENROLL

To enroll in the Radiologic Clinics of North America Continuing Medical Education program, call customer service at 1-800-654-2452 or sign up online at http://www.theclinics.com/home/cme. The CME program is available to subscribers for an additional annual fee USD 245.

Radiologic Clinics of North America

THE CLINICS ARE NOW AVAILABLE ONLINE!

Access your subscription at:
www.theclinics.com

Preface
Imaging of Incidentalomas

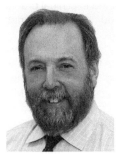

Alec J. Megibow, MD, MPH
Guest Editor

It may be hard for some readers to imagine that cross sectional imaging used to be considered a "special procedure". Now it is the standard of imaging and is the grist of general radiology. This technologic shift has benefitted countless patients. Clinical adaptation of cross-sectional imaging speeds workups, leads to more rapid and informed therapeutic decision-making, and allows noninvasive monitoring of treatments. One needs look no further than the revolution in the treatment of trauma patients or monitoring chemotherapy in lymphoma patients. Yet, as with anything, these great advances have come with a price. This issue considers one of these costs, the incidental lesion, also called the "incidentaloma."

A useful definition for incidental findings comes from D.S. Davis in the *Journal Medicine and Philosophy* in 2007. An incidental finding is "unsought information generated in the seeking of the information one desires." This definition is easily adaptable to imaging. Although unsought information may be beneficial to patients, such as when unsuspected tumors, aneurysms, silent hydronephrosis, stones, etc are serendipitously detected, just as frequently (maybe even more so) the unsought information (the incidentaloma) is detrimental. Patients are subjected to excessive workups, cost, and interventions not to mention excruciating anxiety. The economic impact directly linked to overdiagnosis of incidentalomas has been proven to be a key impediment toward expansion of coverage for CT colonography. They are also a major source of requests for additional imaging. Because these lesions are more frequently insignificant, continued cataloguing of them in radiology report after radiology report without a rational basis on which a clinical recommendation can be made has eroded the credibility of radiologists; individual radiologists will often make disparate recommendations for immediate or long-term follow-up of the same finding. Often these differences are exposed within the same group or department, leaving referring physicians and patients frustrated. Some have even gone so far as to recommend that radiologists' recommendations of follow-up imaging for incidental findings are the equivalent of "self-referral."[1] The problem is further exacerbated by the increasing distancing of referring physicians from interpreting radiologists, particularly in those situations in which the output measure of quality service is turn-around time, where the interpreting radiologist can no longer have direct conversations with the clinicians charged with caring for the patient.

There is a clear need for some level of a rational baseline whereby radiologists can find some level of guidance when they encounter an incidentaloma on an imaging study. This issue of *Radiologic Clinics of North America* is an attempt to be a first step toward organizing a knowledge base that will answer this need specifically for imagers. I have been fortunate in being able to solicit the contributions of a group of thoughtful and experienced radiologists to tackle this problem. The nucleus of the volume stems from the work of the Incidental Findings Committee. This group was

Radiol Clin N Am 49 (2011) xi–xii
doi:10.1016/j.rcl.2011.01.001

organized by Dr Lincoln Berland in his role as Chair of the Body Imaging Committee of the American College of Radiology. Dr Berland reviews the case of the problems caused by incidental lesions, the genesis of the committee, and how the work proceeded toward generation of a white paper that appeared in October 2010 *Journal of American College of Radiology* (JACR). Reports of the four subcommittees are presented. This volume allows more detail to be incorporated into the discussions of individual reports, and readers can get a deeper understanding of the thought processes that created the guidelines that appeared in JACR. Additionally, I have been fortunate to receive contributions from Drs Jeffery Alpert and David Naidich at NYU reviewing not only Fleischner criteria for lung nodules but also for tackling incidentalomas throughout the thorax; Sameer Ahmed working with Karen Horton and Elliott Fishman from Johns Hopkins reviewed the spleen; and Bidyut Pramanik, also from NYU, examined incidentalomas in the nervous system. There are two other unique contributions to this issue: first, Leonard Berlin has written an article about legal ramifications of incidental findings, and second, Pari Pandharipande from the MGH Institute for Technology Assessment has provided an economic analysis of the problems with these lesions.

As stated above, this volume collects the "best thinking" on this controversial topic as of Spring 2011. It is likely that every reader will have first-hand knowledge of cases that do not follow proposed guidelines. However, based on the vast experience of the authors, many cases will be appropriately diagnosed using these guidelines as a basis for decision-making. Also, as these guidelines become established in clinical practice, they will likely be refined and appropriately updated.

In conclusion, I would like to thank the following: Lincoln Berland, who, at the time this project was conceived, was consumed with the editing of the now published white paper; Frank Miller, Consulting Editor for *Radiologic Clinics*, who thought I might be an appropriate choice as editor; and Barton Dudlick and the staff at Elsevier, who provided efficient, seamless, and highly competent editorial services.

Alec J. Megibow, MD, MPH
Department of Radiology
NYU-Langone Medical Center
550 First Avenue
HCC 232
New York, NY 10016, USA

E-mail address:
Alec.Megibow@nyumc.org

REFERENCE

1. Blaivas M, Lyon M. Frequency of radiology self-referral in abdominal computed tomographic scans and the implied cost. Am J Emerg Med 2007;25(4): 396–9.

The American College of Radiology Strategy for Managing Incidental Findings on Abdominal Computed Tomography

Lincoln L. Berland, MD

KEYWORDS
- Computed tomography • Incidental findings • Committee
- Recommendations

BACKGROUND: NEED FOR INCIDENTAL FINDINGS PROJECT

Incidental findings on radiographic studies have been available since the origin of diagnostic radiology. The discovery of such findings was often accepted as simply an unwanted, but unavoidable, byproduct of an important test. With the advent of cross-sectional imaging, the discovery of such findings became more frequent, and their recognition was usually believed to be beneficial by leading to early detection of subclinical disease, and probably to better outcomes.[1–3] However, in recent years, incidentalomas have generated heightened concern and even alarm.[4,5]

It is important to understand the meaning of the term incidental finding. An incidentaloma, as it is also known, may be defined as "An incidentally discovered mass or lesion, detected by CT, MRI, or other imaging modality performed for an unrelated reason."[6] Essentially, these masses or lesions represent findings that are detected but are unrelated to the primary objectives of the examinations.[7–10] However, many such incidental findings are of little importance because they are immediately recognized as unrelated to any condition that would threaten the patient's health. For example, an anomalous retroaortic left renal vein is a common anatomic variant. Many patients have findings indicating prior surgery or trauma but are unlikely to have any acute clinical significance. Although these findings may warrant reporting because they could affect future surgical planning or potentially be mistaken for more important abnormalities, they are not the subject of the remainder of this discussion.

There are several reasons why incidentalomas have evolved from a perceived advantage to a perceived problem. The frequency of incidental findings has markedly increased. The number of computed tomographic (CT) examinations performed in the United States skyrocketed from an estimated 21 million in 1998 to 61 million in 2006, which resulted in several factors, including self-referral by nonradiologists. As has been shown by several studies, nonradiologists tend to refer their patients for more radiographic tests when they have a direct or indirect financial interest in the revenue from the sites to which they refer.[11]

Another cost concern is that some radiologists see the identification of incidentalomas as an opportunity to increase referral business for CT, magnetic resonance (MR) imaging, or other expensive radiological tests, providing financial benefit in a fee-for-service environment that incentivizes increased workload.[12,13]

Department of Radiology, University of Alabama at Birmingham, 619 South 19th Street, N348, Birmingham, AL 35249, USA
E-mail address: lberland@gmail.com

Radiol Clin N Am 49 (2011) 237–243
doi:10.1016/j.rcl.2010.10.003
0033-8389/11/$ — see front matter © 2011 Elsevier Inc. All rights reserved.

Another reason for the increased frequency of incidental findings is that the spatial and contrast resolution of CT has improved substantially over the past 10 to 15 years. Therefore, incidental findings may be more likely to be observed on any single examination as well because many more CT scans are being performed. There has also been a markedly increased awareness of the costs of medical care, which has been associated with heightened political pressure to limit these costs. The increase in the use of CT itself has led to CT becoming a target of regulators and insurers. For example, in many regions, health insurers have implemented preauthorization for CT, MR imaging, and other expensive medical tests. Depending on the location and the insurer, this practice has measurably limited the approval for CT examinations, causing the use of this technique to decline or at least level off in number.[14] Nevertheless, this leveling off is still occurring at a rate higher than just 10 years ago.

The concern about incidental findings has also gradually increased because of support by many for using CT for screening for conditions such as lung cancer and colon polyps. For example, CT colonography has raised the concern among insurers and the federal government that its use, and therefore costs, will increase. The Center for Medicare and Medicaid Services, in a decision memorandum, indicated that one of the reasons that they were declining to approve CT colonography for screening for colon polyps in the Medicare population was the concern that the pursuit of extracolonic findings would substantially increase cost with uncertain benefits.[15]

Because of the paucity of data regarding the importance of reporting and following up incidental findings and the paucity of guidance for managing such findings, there is marked inconsistency in the approach to such findings. One of the few studies in which the performance of multiple experienced radiologists was tested regarding the reporting of incidental findings suggested only modest agreement.[16] There were substantial disagreements in this blinded study regarding both the detection of these findings and the beliefs regarding their need to be further evaluated. In addition, anecdotally, many primary care physicians and other clinicians have found that pursuing incidental findings has come to occupy more of their time and has distracted them from attending to activities that could provide greater benefits. Also, determining how to manage such findings can be confusing for referring physicians unless specific guidance is offered by the interpreting physician.

The fear of medicolegal consequences from underreporting incidental findings has been cited

as an important source of requests for evaluating or following them. Because of the uncertainty about the importance of many of such findings, performing extra tests follows a philosophy of "better safe than sorry." In addition, reinforcing this perception is a prevalent belief within the medical culture itself, particularly within the United States, that medical uncertainty is unacceptable, especially because now there are more sophisticated tests to decrease that uncertainty.[17,18] However, with the limited information currently available and the great array of diagnostic possibilities, it is virtually impossible to calculate the probability that a given finding (eg, a mildly increased attenuation 2-cm liver lesion on a noncontrast CT examination) is likely to represent the early manifestation of a disease for which early intervention could improve the outcome.

The level of experience of readers as well as their philosophy is also likely to influence the nature and frequency of recommendations of the physician interpreting the CT study for additional studies, although the nature and magnitude of this effect is unclear. It is a common experience among academic body-imaging radiologists to encounter an excessive number of recommendations for further studies from radiology residents, who understandably do not have the experience to conclusively characterize incidental findings or appreciate their importance (or lack thereof). At the other end of the spectrum, highly experienced academic subspecialists in tertiary referral centers have often encountered cases in which initially subtle findings led to serious medical consequences. These findings heighten their concern and perhaps even falsely elevate their perception of the probability that an incidental finding encountered in a similar situation may be important. Again, although these effects of such differences in experience are unclear, it is highly probable that the level of experience of the interpreter plays a substantial role in the approach that radiologists take to how they report and make recommendations for managing incidentalomas.

COSTS AND CONSEQUENCES OF MANAGING INCIDENTAL FINDINGS

Supporting all these concerns are anecdotal observations and some retrospective and prospective studies on the benefits and costs of working up or following incidental findings. Among the largest populations of patients who have been studied for incidental findings are patients undergoing CT colonography for screening, for failed colonoscopy, or for symptoms or other medical findings suspicious for colonic disease.[7,10] There is a wide variation in the projected costs of following such findings and there is little data to suggest how detecting and following such findings have affected outcome.

One example of the difficulty in understanding these effects is renal cell carcinoma (RCC). This condition has increased markedly in incidence since the advent of cross-sectional imaging, with about 61% of all cases of RCC being detected incidentally on CT scans performed for another indication. However, the overall death rate from RCC has changed little, despite a marked increase in early detection.

One of the reasons for this apparent discrepancy is the problem of overdiagnosis,[19,20] which is the occurrence of histologically confirmed cancerous masses, for which their natural behavior is unknown. Statistics suggest that in many cases, such cancers would never become symptomatic or clinically apparent in another way or would never cause the patient's life span or health to be altered. These cancers are commonly termed as those that "you would die with, rather than die from." For example, although approximately 0.5% of all patients die of RCC, studies suggest that RCC is found in as many as 2% of all autopsies. The problem is that when these masses are biopsied or removed and cancer is diagnosed histologically, it is not known which of them represent cancers that would grow to become symptomatic or to metastasize and which would remain indolent and asymptomatic. Therefore, by necessity, all such cancers must be treated as if they were potentially fatal. This problem of overdiagnosis is found not only with renal cancers but also with breast, lung, prostate, and thyroid cancers as well as other conditions.

Although it is a common public perception that early detection of disease, before the onset of symptoms, is highly desirable, it depends greatly on both the specific condition and at what stage the disease is detected. For example, there is no available data suggesting that early detection of lymphoma affects outcome. Detecting metastatic cancer of many types before the onset of symptoms is also unlikely to change the course of disease. Multiple attempts to achieve early detection of ovarian cancer with imaging has suggested that finding it at both an asymptomatic and curable stage with imaging is exceedingly difficult.[21,22]

Considerations of costs cannot be limited to the costs of the extra tests performed alone. In many cases, these tests have potential side effects and may lead to more invasive and risky procedures, such as biopsies or surgery. Naturally, in a small number of cases, complications from these procedures occur, which may lead to very high costs. A phenomenon termed "cascade syndrome" occurs in which one examination may lead to one or multiple incidental findings, which in turn lead to multiple other examinations and procedures sequentially. One example of this phenomenon was published in the *journal Radiology*,[23] described by the former Chairman of the Department of Radiology at Emory University as having occurred to himself. The investigator underwent a CT colonography; had renal, hepatic, and lung masses detected; and underwent additional CT scans, a positron emission tomography scan, a liver biopsy, and a video-aided thoracoscopy with wedge resection. He experienced excruciating postoperative pain, 5 weeks of recuperation, and charges more than $50,000. Fortunately, all findings were benign.

Another difficulty in interpreting the benefits from detecting disease before the onset of symptoms is that this detection may lead to a false impression of increased longevity. The period of detection before the onset of symptoms may be added to the overall survival time, suggesting that early detection has been beneficial. This phenomenon is termed "length bias."

Many believe that the value of early detection is primarily in the early detection of cancer. However, at least one study using a Monte Carlo simulation technique, suggests that most of the benefit may be in the early detection of abdominal aortic aneurysms (AAAs).[24] Although ruptured AAAs represent a relatively small percentage of total deaths, the value of early detection of AAAs is high because they are usually asymptomatic, and treatment with surgical bypass or endostent placement is highly effective in reducing deaths.[25]

FORMATION OF THE INCIDENTAL FINDINGS COMMITTEE OF THE AMERICAN COLLEGE OF RADIOLOGY

In 2005, I was appointed as the Chair of the Committee on Body Imaging under the Body Imaging Commission (at that time under the leadership of Dr N. Reed Dunnick) of the American College of Radiology (ACR). One of the core responsibilities of this committee is the development and ongoing review and revision of radiological guidelines documents in multiple areas. Because I began to hear presentations at national meetings from radiology leaders such as Dr Richard Gore and others on incidental findings in the abdomen, this helped reinforce my perception from my own busy academic practice that such incidental findings had not received adequate attention. I also appreciated from my participation in these guidelines reviews awareness of the ACR Appropriateness Guidelines and from the efforts of organizations such as the Fleischner Society (which released guidelines for managing pulmonary nodules in 2005[26]) that an effort to generate a consensus on managing incidental findings on abdominal imaging could also be valuable.

In 2006, with the support of Dr Dunnick and the ACR, we organized an Incidental Findings Committee under the Body Imaging Commission, which is now led by Dr James A. Brink. We were able to assemble a group of thought leaders within radiology to address this problem, and we began to contemplate how such an effort could be organized and what its objectives would be. We agreed that there were little data on how incidental findings should be reported and managed and agreed that some method of consensus development would be a reasonable objective. In addition, the committee believed that although the primary product of the committee would be practical guidance for radiologists for managing incidental findings, other objectives might also be desirable, which included the development of common terminology and providing baseline parameters and recommendations for researchers to test.

PROCESS OF DEVELOPING RECOMMENDATIONS

Although it was believed that using a modified Delphi technique (such as used for the ACR Appropriateness Criteria) might be worthwhile, after discussion among the committee members and representatives of the ACR, it was concluded that such an approach might not be applicable to this effort and would require resources not available to us. Additional discussions occurred regarding whether physicians outside radiology would be included in this effort. It was agreed that acceptability of recommendations that might come from this committee was likely to be enhanced by the participation of nonradiologists. However, after considering this option, the committee agreed that to include nonradiologists would be difficult and time consuming and might also hinder progress by requiring the review and approval of nonradiology subspecialty professional organizations. Therefore, although considered important, we agreed that the involvement of nonradiologists should be deferred until the committee had produced its initial set of recommendations.

As the Chair of the Renal Subcommittee, Dr Stuart Silverman decided to approach the task of developing recommendations by developing an article reviewing and summarizing the available literature, which was completed and published in the *journal Radiology*.[27] This article provided the basis for the final recommendations released in the ACR Incidental Findings Committee White Paper.[28] Although this project was initiated within the ACR, multiple organizations have an interest in incidental findings in the abdomen. Therefore, in addition to the ACR, the Society of Computed Body Tomography and Magnetic Resonance (SCBT-MR), the Society of Gastrointestinal Radiology (SGR), and the Society of Uroradiology (SUR) were consulted. Most members of the committee are fellows or members of more than one of these organizations. Through the involvement of these societies, it was hoped that once recommendations were developed, the societies would actively endorse and assist in disseminating these recommendations.

Unfortunately, the progress of the committee was initially slow because of several obstacles of commitment and support and extended deliberations regarding the appropriate methods with which to proceed. However, in mid-2008, the issue of the potential approval of CT colonography for widespread reimbursement was attracting increased attention. It had already been perceived that the concern about the implications regarding incidental findings could potentially affect decisions in this area. At about this time, Dr James A. Brink assumed the leadership of the Body Imaging Commission. The concern about the effect of incidentalomas on CT colonography was expressed by Dr Elizabeth McFarland as the Chair of the ACR CT Colonography Committee and subsequently Dr Judy Yee, who succeeded as the Chair of this committee. All agreed that the effort to develop recommendations on incidental findings should be prioritized and accelerated.

WHITE PAPER TO COMMUNICATE RECOMMENDATIONS

If the committee were to develop formal guidelines analogous to the ACR Appropriateness Criteria, it would require a lengthy review and approval process by the ACR. Therefore, the commissioner, representatives of the ACR, and the committee agreed that the most efficient vehicle for codifying and disseminating guidance on incidental findings is a white paper.

Among the challenges facing the development of these recommendations was the concern that these recommendations should be broadly acceptable, easy to access, and straightforward to understand and apply. To accomplish this objective, it was agreed that the white paper should illustrate recommendations in the form of tables or flowcharts, supported by more detailed text. Such tables proved difficult to construct, and the committee eventually decided to develop flowcharts. These flowcharts were patterned after flowcharts developed for managing incidental adrenal masses designed by Dr Boland and colleagues.[29]

The large potential scope of the project also required that the effort be narrowed. The organ systems that may contain incidental findings include the kidneys, liver, adrenal glands, pancreas, aorta, spleen, lymph nodes, gallbladder, biliary system, ovaries, and others. To optimize value, while keeping the task manageable, the committee decided to address the 4 organs with the largest number of potentially important incidental findings, the kidneys, liver, adrenal glands, and pancreas.

Also, to assure that the submission of the white paper is not excessively delayed, it was investigated whether the article could be submitted under the auspices of the ACR without having to go through the formal approval process of the college. It was determined that publishing such a white paper was acceptable, provided it was not claimed to represent formal guidelines or other type of formal statement of the ACR.

DISSEMINATING THE WHITE PAPER AND ENCOURAGING ITS USE

Among the core advantages of adopting these recommendations is the improved consistency of the approach among various practitioners. It has been well demonstrated in many environments in medicine and business that quality is enhanced by decreasing variations of practice. Therefore, it is hoped that by broadly distributing this scheme for managing incidental findings, greater uniformity can be achieved.

This article[28] has been published in the *Journal of the American College of Radiology*. Based on the participation of the ACR, the SCBT-MR, the SGR, and the SUR, these societies are being requested to actively endorse and promote the use of these recommendations to their membership. We also hope to increase awareness of this white paper through articles in appropriate newsletters and Web sites. We expect this work to attract attention and hope to solicit both positive and constructive critical comments to help refine these recommendations and possibly modify the process of their development.

POSSIBLE FUTURE TASKS FOR THE COMMITTEE
Improving Accessibility and Usability

Even when radiologists become aware of these recommendations, facilitating their integration into practice is challenging. Distilling this management scheme into flowcharts is intended to make this guidance more accessible and usable. It is hoped that in addition to having the entire white paper available near workstations, it is expected that the flowcharts will be printed and posted for easy reference. We will also encourage the participating societies to place links on their Web sites to the white paper or post other summary materials as we prepare them.

The complexity of these subjects makes even the graphic representation of the management scheme potentially confusing. Therefore, one consideration is to attempt to summarize recommendations in other formats that can be accessed online or provide a reorganized structured Web-based method to access the recommendations for patients.

Soliciting Comments and Formalizing the Process of Developing Recommendations

As discussed, this white paper is not intended to be a final document but a step in an evolving process. We will evaluate comments from users but also plan to enroll other interested clinical physicians in the process of revision. For example, we would expect to include nephrologists and urologists in addressing renal masses, hepatologists for liver masses, and so forth. At some point, it might also be reasonable to solicit the opinions and endorsement of nonradiology specialty societies. How the inclusion of nonradiologists proceeds will partly depend on the resources available through the ACR and other involved radiology societies.

Another avenue for promoting the use of these recommendations and guidance would be to attempt to acquire the formal approval of the ACR. As part of this effort, the ACR may wish to establish a specific consensus technology, such as the modified Delphi technique used for the ACR Appropriateness Criteria.

Although the white paper addresses several of the key organ systems in which incidental findings are found, there are many other potential types of incidental findings. These findings include ovarian cystic masses, lymphadenopathy, biliary dilation, abdominal aortic and other aneurysms, various gastrointestinal findings, and others. The committee, or another group, may wish to tackle such findings.

Encouraging Research to Test Our Recommendations

As noted, one of the core problems in managing incidental findings is the severe paucity of scientific research on the nature and natural history of these findings. The committee is well aware of the gaps and potential flaws in the approach we have proposed. One of the often-repeated desires of the committee has been that our efforts result in further research. We believe that by disseminating our recommendations for specific management approaches based on specific mass sizes and characteristics, researchers could test the parameters we propose for their efficacy. In addition, we believe that providing this structure for studying this problem could also help encourage various organizations to materially support research in this area.

SUMMARY

There has been a dramatically increased awareness of the substantial clinical challenges posed by incidental findings found on cross-sectional imaging. We believe that the efforts of the ACR Incidental Findings Committee are advancing the ability to create a consistent and rational approach to these findings. However, the committee also appreciates that our level of knowledge about the importance of these findings and how to appropriately manage them remains embryonic, and we are prepared to keep this issue in the consciousness of medical professionals and to assist in furthering knowledge about incidental findings.

REFERENCES

1. Hara AK, Johnson CD, MacCarty RL, et al. Incidental extracolonic findings at CT colonography. Radiology 2000;215:353–7.
2. Gluecker TM, Johnson CD, Wilson LA, et al. Extracolonic findings at CT colonography: evaluation of prevalence and cost in a screening population. Gastroenterology 2003;124:911–6.
3. Tolan DJ, Armstrong EM, Chapman AH. Replacing barium enema with CT colonography in patients older than 70 years: the importance of detecting extracolonic abnormalities. AJR Am J Roentgenol 2007;189:1104–11.
4. Fletcher RH, Pignone M. Extracolonic findings with computed tomographic colonography: asset or liability? Arch Intern Med 2008;168(7):685–6.
5. Berland LL. Incidental extracolonic findings on CT colonography: the impending deluge and its implications. J Am Coll Radiol 2009;6(1):14–20.
6. The Free Dictionary by Farlex, Inc. Available at: http://medical-dictionary.thefreedictionary.com/Incidental+finding. Accessed May 15, 2010.
7. Pickhardt PJ, Hanson ME, Vanness DJ, et al. Unsuspected extracolonic findings at screening CT colonography: clinical and economic impact. Radiology 2008;249(1):151–9.
8. Bovio S, Cataldi A, Reimondo G, et al. Prevalence of adrenal incidentaloma in a contemporary computerized tomography series. J Endocrinol Invest 2006;29(4):298–302.
9. Wagner SC, Morrison WB, Carrino JA, et al. Picture archiving and communication system: effect on reporting of incidental findings. Radiology 2002;225(2):500–5.
10. Yee J, Kumar NN, Godara S, et al. Extracolonic abnormalities discovered incidentally at CT colonography in a male population. Radiology 2005;236(2):519–26.
11. Levin DC, Rao VM. Turf wars in radiology: updated evidence on the relationship between self-referral and the overutilization of imaging. J Am Coll Radiol 2008;5(7):806–10.
12. Blaivas M, Lyon M. Frequency of radiology self-referral in abdominal computed tomographic scans and the implied cost. Am J Emerg Med 2007;25:396–9.
13. Sistrom CL, Dreyer KJ, Dang PP, et al. Recommendations for additional imaging in radiology reports: multifactorial analysis of 5.9 million examinations. Radiology 2009;253(2):453–61.
14. Levin DC, Bree RL, Rao VM, et al. A prior authorization program of a radiology Benefits management company and how it has affected utilization of advanced diagnostic imaging. J Am Coll Radiol 2010;7(1):33–8.
15. Centers for Medicare and Medicaid Services. Decision memo for screening computed tomography colonography (CTC) for colorectal cancer (CAG-00396N). Available at: http://www.cms.gov/medicare-coverage-database/details/nca-decision-memo.aspx?NCAId=220&ver=13&NcaName=Screening+Computed+Tomography+Colonography+%28CTC%29+for+Colorectal+Cancer&TAId=58&IsPopup=y&AspxAuto DetectCookieSupport=1&bc=AAAAAAAAEAAA&. Accessed November 26, 2010.
16. Obuchowski NA, Holden D, Modic MT, et al. Total-body screening: preliminary results of a pilot randomized controlled trial. J Am Coll Radiol 2007;4:604–11.
17. Elstein AS. On the origins and development of evidence-based medicine and medical decision making. Inflamm Res 2004;53(Suppl 2):S184–9.
18. Wolf SM, Lawrenz FP, Nelson CA, et al. Managing incidental findings in human subjects research: analysis and recommendations. J Law Med Ethics 2008;36(2):219–48, 211.

19. Fenton JJ, Weiss NS, Black WC. Screening computed tomography: will it result in overdiagnosis of renal carcinoma? Cancer 2004;100(5):986–90.

20. Black WC. Overdiagnosis: an under recognized cause of confusion and harm in cancer screening. J Natl Cancer Inst 2000;92:1280–2.

21. Van Nagell Jr, DePriest PD, Reedy MB, et al. The efficacy of transvaginal sonographic screening in asymptomatic women at risk for ovarian carcinoma. Gynecol Oncol 2000;77:350–6.

22. Sato S, Yokoyama Y, Sakamoto T, et al. Usefulness of mass screening for ovarian carcinoma using transvaginal ultrasonography. Cancer 2000;89:582–8.

23. Casarella WJ. A patient's viewpoint on a current controversy. Radiology 2002;224(3):927.

24. Hassan C, Pickhardt P, Laghi A, et al. Computed tomographic colonography to screen for colorectal cancer, extracolonic cancer, and aortic aneurysm: model simulation with cost effectiveness analysis. Arch Intern Med 2008;168:696–705.

25. Wilmink AB, Quick CR, Hubbard CS, et al. Effectiveness and cost of screening for abdominal aortic aneurysm: results of a population screening program. J Vasc Surg 2003;38:72–7.

26. MacMahon H, Austin JH, Gamsu G, et al. Guidelines for management of small pulmonary nodules detected on CT scans: a statement from the Fleischner Society. Radiology 2005;237(2): 395–400.

27. Silverman SG, Israel GM, Herts BR, et al. Management of the incidental renal mass. Radiology 2008; 249(1):16–31.

28. Berland LL, Silverman SG, Gore RM, et al. Managing incidental findings on abdominal CT: white paper of the ACR Incidental Findings Committee. J Am Coll Radiol 2010;7:754–73.

29. Boland GW, Blake MA, Hahn PF, et al. Incidental adrenal lesions: principles, techniques, and algorithms for imaging characterization. Radiology 2008;249(3):756–75.

The Incidentaloma: A Medicolegal Dilemma

Leonard Berlin, MD[a,b,*]

KEYWORDS

- Incidentalomas • Malpractice • Medicolegal

THE CASES

Case 1

In October 2006, an 83-year-old, small, frail-looking woman, with a history of chronic obstructive pulmonary disease and smoking a pack of cigarettes daily for the previous 50 years, visited her family internist with complaints of cough and shortness of breath. Her physician referred her to the outpatient radiology department of a local hospital, where on October 19, 2006 she underwent posterior-anterior and lateral chest radiographies. A radiologist interpreted the examination as disclosing "evidence of chronic obstructive pulmonary disease with scattered fibrotic changes, but otherwise essentially normal study."

Ten months later the patient, now complaining of increasing cough and chest discomfort, again underwent chest radiography on the order of her family physician. A different radiologist interpreted the examination as disclosing a "2 cm mass in the right mid-lung field, suspicious for malignancy." Computed tomography (CT) confirmed the finding, and a subsequent biopsy disclosed non–small cell carcinoma. Despite chemotherapy, the patient developed numerous metastases and died on July 17, 2008.

A short time after the diagnosis was established, the patient's physician informed the patient and her husband that in reviewing the earlier radiographs taken in October, 2006 with a radiologist, it was discovered that a small nodule had been present in the right midlung field, but no mention of it had been made in the radiographic report. Soon thereafter, the patient and her family filed a medical malpractice lawsuit against the radiologist who had interpreted the chest radiographs taken in 2006, alleging that his missing of the small lung cancer caused a delay in diagnosis such that the patient was prevented from obtaining curative treatment.

During discovery proceedings, the defendant radiologist testified that he had initially observed a small nodule of less than 1 cm diameter in the fifth anterior interspace of the patient's right lung but that he decided to not mention the finding in his report because he felt "certain" that the density was a nipple shadow. An expert radiology witness for the plaintiff testified that it would be most unusual to have a unilateral nipple shadow, and furthermore, if the defendant radiologist had suspected that the density was a nipple shadow, "he should have had another film taken with a metal marker placed on the woman's nipple." An expert radiology witness retained by the defense testified that the appearance of the nodule on the earlier chest radiograph was very typical of a nipple shadow and as for it being on one side only, referred to a radiology textbook that stated that "Nipple shadows are typically bilateral, although in some cases only a single nipple shadow is seen on frontal radiographs."[1] Adding that it was not necessary for the defendant radiologist to suggest additional radiographs with a metal marker on the patient's nipple, the defense expert referred to another radiology textbook that stated, "A film with metallic nipple markers may occasionally be necessary to differentiate a nipple shadow from an intrapulmonary lesion"[2]; the expert placed great emphasis on the words "occasionally may be necessary."

[a] Department of Radiology, Rush Medical College, 1653 West Congress Parkway, Chicago, IL 60612, USA
[b] Department of Radiology, NorthShore University HealthSystem, Skokie Hospital, 9600 Gross Point Road, Skokie, IL 60076, USA
* Department of Radiology, NorthShore University HealthSystem, Skokie Hospital, 9600 Gross Point Road, Skokie, IL 60076.
E-mail address: lberlin@live.com

Radiol Clin N Am 49 (2011) 245–255
doi:10.1016/j.rcl.2010.11.002

The lawsuit eventually went to trial before a judge, who ruled in favor of the patient.

Case 2

A 45-year-old woman was referred by her family physician to an otolaryngologist because of repeated episodes of sinusitis. Over the previous 3 years, the patient had undergone 5 CT examinations of the paranasal sinuses, all of which had been interpreted by the same radiologist as disclosing varying degrees of sinusitis, ranging from acute disease to almost normal findings. Nonetheless, despite intermittent antibiotic and decongestant treatment, the patient did not make any permanent progress in controlling her recurring infection.

After examining the patient and reviewing the previous radiological studies, the otolaryngologist recommended surgery. During the surgical procedure, the otolaryngologist discovered a small dentigerous cyst just above 2 of the patient's molar teeth, encroaching on but not eroding the floor of the maxillary sinus. Soon after surgery was completed, the otolaryngologist reviewed all of the radiological images with the patient and her husband, pointing out that the dentigerous cyst had been present but unreported on all 5 studies. Although the cyst had not changed significantly in size, nevertheless in the opinion of the otolaryngologist, it had represented a major causative factor in the patient's sinusitis having been refractory to antibiotic treatment.

The patient subsequently filed a malpractice lawsuit against the radiologist who had interpreted the sinus CT studies. An expert radiology witness for the plaintiff testified in a discovery deposition that the dentigerous cyst was obvious and should have been diagnosed by the defendant radiologist. The defendant radiologist testified that he had seen a very small dentigerous cyst on each of the 5 sinus CT studies but had felt it was simply an incidental finding, which had no bearing on the patient's recurring chronic sinusitis. An expert radiology witness retained by the defense supported the opinion of the defendant radiologist. "The cyst did not change in size or configuration over a five-year period, is essentially a dental problem, did not erode the boney floor of the maxillary sinus, and thus had no effect on the patient's sinusitis," contended the defense expert.

The case proceeded to trial, at the conclusion of which the jury rendered a verdict in favor of the defendant radiologist.

INCIDENTALOMAS

Clinicians ordinarily have at least one and perhaps several potential diagnoses in mind when they request radiological examinations in a patient. Generally, these impressions or at least the patients' history, symptoms, or laboratory tests that raise the possibility of certain diagnoses are transmitted to the radiologist who is interpreting the radiological examination, and generally the radiologist includes in the report a reference to the clinician's concerns. On occasion, the radiologist notes a finding in a radiological study which is totally unrelated to the clinician's reasons for requesting the radiological examination, that is, a finding that is incidentally noted, an incidentaloma. Both the medical malpractice lawsuits briefly summarized in the opening paragraphs of this article focused on incidentalomas, a tiny lung nodule thought by the radiologist to represent a nipple shadow on a chest radiograph and a small dentigerous cyst felt to be of no clinical significance on a paranasal sinus CT scan. In both these cases, the interpreting radiologists believed that the incidentalomas were sufficiently medically unimportant that there was no need to mention their existence in the radiological reports. And in both cases, medical malpractice lawsuits were filed. These cases lead us to rhetorically ask whether every incidentaloma noted by every radiologist on every radiological study should be noted and documented in every radiological written report. In this article this question is analyzed from 2 perspectives, the legal and the ethical.

The Legal Perspective

Nearly a century ago in an often-quoted New York Appeals Court decision, Justice Benjamin Cardozo proclaimed, "Any human being of adult years and sound mind has a right to determine what shall be done with his own body."[3] A quarter of a century ago a federal appeals court held that, "A physician undertaking an examination has a duty to disclose what he had found and to warn the examinee of any finding that would indicate the patient is in any danger." Fifteen years ago, in referring to a radiologist's interpretation of radiographs, an Ohio Appeals Court stated, "As part of the duty the physician must reveal to the patient that which in his best interest he should know. The radiologist must share liability if he has failed in adequately communicating the diagnosis to the attending physician."[4]

The 3 court pronouncements just cited dealt with relatively significant abnormalities. Some incidentalomas indeed represent significant medical abnormalities, but many other incidentalomas are quite equivocal as to their clinical significance. No radiologist would question the need to report what is believed to be a clinically significant incidentaloma and thus a medical malpractice lawsuit related to such a report would be extremely rare. However, as already seen, a radiologist's failure to report what is believed to be an incidentaloma of equivocal or no clinical significance may well have medical-legal ramifications.

Is the Incidentaloma a Granuloma or a Carcinoma, Giving the Jury a Tune It can Whistle

Case 3

A 66-year-old woman was admitted to the hospital for treatment of a right lower quadrant abscess secondary to perforation of the appendix. During her hospitalization, multiple CT scans of the patient's abdomen and pelvis were obtained and interpreted accurately by 2 radiologist members of the hospital's radiology group. Both radiologists included in their abdominal and pelvic CT reports a statement that read, "Incidental finding includes a calcified granuloma in the right lung base." The patient recovered from her abdominal illness, but 1 year later was diagnosed with a right lower lobe lung carcinoma. A malpractice lawsuit was lodged against the 2 radiologists, alleging that because the pulmonary calcification was surrounded by a minimal soft tissue density, they should have raised the question of carcinoma on the CT scans. The lawsuit proceeded to a jury trial. The first defendant radiologist was called to the witness stand and questioned by the plaintiff's attorney:

Q: Doctor, when you issue a report that a mass in the lung is nothing to worry about, you would expect that the doctor reading that report would rely on it and would therefore probably not do anything more to try to figure out if that mass in the lung is cancer, do you agree?

A: Yes.

Q: And would you say that before you issue a report that a mass in the lung is nothing to worry about, you owe it to the patient to be mighty sure of what you are saying?

A: Yes.

Q: Would you agree that when a CT scan shows a lung mass, the fact that the mass contains calcium does not always allow you to conclude that the mass is benign?

A: Yes.

Q: Doctor, it is recognized, is it not, that you can have a calcified granuloma with nice smooth borders, and then a malignancy can grow around the granuloma and create edges, correct?

A: It can happen, but it is very rare.

Q: Doctor, I didn't ask if it's rare, I asked only if it is recognized that a malignancy can grow around a granuloma? Answer the question yes or no.

A: Yes.

Q: Doctor, is it not true that there are three ways in which you might report your conclusions concerning a lung mass: benign, which is what you did; indeterminate, which means it has characteristics that might make it malignant, or might not make it malignant, you don't know; and suspicious for malignancy?

A: Yes.

Q: Doctor, when a lung mass shown on a radiology study is indeterminate, is it true that the standard of practice requires that the radiologist communicate to the attending physician that the mass is indeterminate?

A: Yes.

Q: Doctor, would you agree that when issuing a report that a mass is a benign granuloma, it's probably going to cause the physician receiving the report to engage in no further testing, and that if the mass is cancer, it means that the cancer will continue to grow undetected, and that furthermore, if you issue a report that something is a benign granuloma without being awfully sure of it, that report can be a death sentence for the patient?

A: I suppose that's true.

Q: Doctor, looking at the films, is the calcification in the center of the lesion of is it off-center? Keep in mind that in your report, you called the calcification central.

A: It's central to me.

Q: Well, Doctor, if someone looking at this thought the calcification was closer to the top than the bottom, that's not really in the center, correct?

A: Yes.

Q: Doctor, if this calcification is not in the center, then it's off-center, and therefore you should not have issued your report in the way you did, correct? And if judgments are to be made about whether or not to follow up a lung lesion, is it your responsibility to leave the judgment-making in the hands of the patient and the patient's physician?

A: I was the patient's physician at the time and I used my own judgment.

Q: Well, Doctor, everything we do in life involves judgment. When you are driving down the street and you see a red light, you exercise your judgment whether to stop or go through it, I suppose. If you go through a red light and you injure someone, it's not a defense that you went through that red light in the exercise of your judgment, is it?

A: That would be bad judgment, correct.

Q: That would be negligent judgment?

A: Yes.

Q: So just because one is exercising judgment doesn't mean that whatever you do is okay, does it, and thus you can be negligent in the exercise of your judgment, can't you?

A: If your judgment is wrong, that's true.

Q: Doctor, can you see how a reasonably well-qualified radiologist looking at this mass, seeing the position of the calcification, and looking at the borders that are irregular, would report this as indeterminate for malignancy?

A: Different people will report it in different ways but I suppose perhaps someone could.

Q: Just not you?

A: Correct.

The plaintiff's lawyer then called the second defendant radiologist to the witness stand.

Q: Doctor, would you agree that if this mass should have been reported as indeterminate for cancer on the first CT, you had the same responsibility to report it the same way on the follow-up CT?

A: If it should have been reported as indeterminate, yes.

Q: Doctor, let's talk about your report of the CT that showed a mass in the lung. If you are going to make a life-and-death decision for a patient it would be a pretty good idea to try to make a decision as to what the borders look like, what the calcification looks like, and whether the calcification is central or eccentric, would it not?

A: Yes.

Q: Doctor, as a radiologist, you do not make a diagnosis of lung cancer, do you? Pathologists do that, right? What you do is like the screeners at the airport. A suitcase comes through the x-ray machine, something shows up, it might be a gun, it might not be a gun, they don't know, so they pull the bag off the line. That's what a radiologist does. And then someone else takes a look in the bag and sometimes it's a gun and sometimes it isn't.

A: Well, I went to a lot more schooling than the people doing what you are saying, and thus I don't think that is a good analogy.

Q: Okay, but what a radiologist does is alert people that there may be a problem in a lung and then those people go on and they make the tests and they do whatever needs to be done to determine if it is truly a problem, right?

A: Yes.

Q: Doctor, is the calcification in this mass eccentric?

A: No, I don't believe so.

Q: Now, Doctor, you were in this courtroom earlier when your partner testified. Did you hear him say that the calcification may be a little bit eccentric?

A: I disagree with that and I disagree with my partner.

Q: Well, Doctor, since you disagree with your partner, it would have been nice to discuss that disagreement when the patient was still in the hospital and could have benefited from it, wouldn't it?

A: Yes.

Q: Doctor, even though the occurrence may be rare, the patient had a right to expect that the radiologist reading her study would know that a lung cancer can engulf a granuloma and create an eccentric calcification, correct?

A: Yes.

Q: Doctor, when you are looking at this mass, and you've got a part of the border that looks benign and a part of the border that looks suspicious, and a calcification that may be central but maybe it's eccentric, then it wouldn't be unreasonable, would it, to allow the patient and the patient's doctor to decide what steps to take next?

A: That's not unreasonable, no.

Q: But, Doctor, when you issue a report that tells them it is a granuloma, that's not going to happen is it?

A: That's correct.

Q: Doctor, with regard to the responsibility that you owe a patient, wouldn't you agree that this responsibility requires that an indeterminate mass be recorded as indeterminate, and that if you fail to report it as indeterminate, you are not only doing the patient a great disservice, but you may be sentencing the patient to death because a malignant process will not be diagnosed when it is still in a curable stage?

A: Yes.

Q: And, furthermore, you have the same duty to the patient regardless of whether the CT is a study of the chest or a study of the abdomen that shows the chest. Isn't that true?

A: Yes.

Q: Doctor, you've told this jury that the only way you can say that the calcification was in the middle of this mass is by disagreeing with your partner.

A: That's true.

Q: In that situation, didn't the patient have a right for the two of you to talk and for the two of you to issue a report that was indeterminate? Wasn't that the patient's right, Doctor?

A: I guess.

Q: And isn't that a right that the patient had pursuant to accepted standards of radiologic practice? Don't the accepted standards of medical practice require that two doctors reading a study who are in a disagreement of what that study shows and who are in the same office together and they are dealing with something that is potentially a life and death situation, don't accepted standards of medical practice require in that situation that the two of you talk? Doesn't the accepted standard of practice require that the two of you get together and try to figure out what this is and how to report it?

A: I can't answer that yes or no.

Q: Doctor, a mass in someone else's lung is a big deal, isn't it? Until you determine whether it's malignant or benign, if someone found a mass in your lung, it would be a big deal wouldn't it, and if so, would it be any less of a big deal in the patient's lung?

A: It would be a big deal.

Q: So you and your partner disagreed on the appearance of this mass. At this point, you knew there was a dispute between you and your associate radiologist. Wouldn't you then agree that the accepted standard of radiologic practice required that the two of you discuss this dispute?

A: No.

Q: No? So, Doctor, in your radiology group, where a patient has two radiology studies done that were read by two different radiologists, and the radiologists disagreed with each other, the standard in your group was not to discuss it, is that what you are saying? Doesn't the standard in your group or in any other radiology group require that where there is a disagreement on the interpretation of a radiology study, it should be discussed?

A: Yes.

Q: And that discussion never happened in this case did it?

A: That discussion never occurred as far as I remember.

Q: That's not a great way to practice medicine or radiology, is it?

The plaintiff's attorney concluded his questioning of the radiologist without waiting for an answer.

In his closing argument, the plaintiff's attorney told the jury that the question before them was whether the calcification was central or eccentric. If the jury felt that the calcification was eccentric, argued the attorney, then the jury had to conclude that the radiologists should have categorized the mass as indeterminate rather than simply as a benign granuloma. The attorney reiterated his earlier claim that had the lesion been called indeterminate, the patient's attending physician would immediately have obtained a biopsy, which in turn would have almost certainly have effected a cure of the patient's lung cancer. Instead, asserted the attorney, the patient was given a death sentence because of the negligent actions of the 2 defendant radiologists.

The plaintiff's attorney then used the analogy of a warning light appearing on the dashboard of a car. "When the warning light appears on your dashboard," said the attorney, "it is in your best interest to go to the mechanic to have the abnormality checked out. The defendant radiologists had a warning light on the dashboard that they ignored."

After deliberation, the jury found that both defendant radiologists had been negligent and awarded the family of the deceased patient $800,000 in damages.[5]

In his book *Damages* that chronicles an actual malpractice lawsuit from its inception to its resolution in a jury trial, Werth[6] wrote

Trials, as any courtroom lawyer knows, are only nominally about law and truth. More often, they are about the personalities and charisma of the lawyers themselves. Trials are a form of theater, and the ability to weave dramatic stories and portray them grippingly in court…to "give the jury a tune it can whistle after the show lets out."

In the lawsuit just described, the plaintiff's attorney did indeed give the jury a "tune it can whistle":

If the calcification was central, the mass was a granuloma,

*But if the calcification was eccentric, then
the mass was a carcinoma;*
    *If the mass was a granuloma, you can set
the radiologists free,*
    *But if the mass was a carcinoma, then you
must find the radiologists guilty.*

An experienced and effective plaintiff's attorney can easily give a jury a similar "tune it can whistle" when a lawsuit centers on the question of whether an incidental radiological finding represented an incidentaloma that need not have been reported because in retrospect it never materialized into any pathologic condition or an incidentaloma that should have been reported because in retrospect it represented an early carcinoma. "If the incidental finding turned out to be a benign incidentaloma, set the radiologist free; but if the incidental finding turned out to be a carcinoma, then find the radiologist guilty." Such a "tune" is eminently successful in a courtroom trial by jury as it was in this particular case because it exploits 2 different biases, hindsight bias and outcome bias.

Hindsight bias and outcome bias

Hindsight bias is defined as "The tendency for people with knowledge of the actual outcome of an event to believe falsely that they would have predicted the outcome."[7] Outcome bias is defined as "The tendency for people to attribute blame more readily when the outcome of an event is serious than when the outcome is comparatively minor."[8] In strictly legal terms, the standard of care for radiologists or nonradiology physicians calls for them to conduct themselves as would reasonable physicians under the same or similar conditions or circumstances as they existed at the time of the event in question. Thus, in strictly legal terms, neither hindsight bias nor outcome bias should play any role whatsoever in a jury's deliberation as to whether a given defendant physician did or did not violate the standard of care under the circumstances that existed at the time the alleged act of malpractice had occurred. The "tune that can be whistled," which obviously encompasses both hindsight and outcome biases, therefore, is not supposed to influence the jury in its deliberation; but from a practical point of view, once jurors hear the "tune," it is difficult if at all possible for them to ignore it.

PREVALENCE OF INCIDENTALOMAS

Incidentalomas in radiological studies are commonplace. Up to 67% of the population in the United States evaluated with ultrasonography have an incidental thyroid nodule, of which 6% to 13% yields malignancy; the majority of these nodules are papillary cancers, which are benign, with a reported 30-year survival of 95% in this population.[9] Pituitary incidentalomas are very common, with a prevalence of up to 20%; most of these need no treatment.[10] Adrenal incidentalomas are common with an extremely low incidence of carcinoma.[11] Nearly 50% of all patients who undergo virtual colonography have incidentalomas, and 7% to 12% of such patients undergo additional testing.[12]

Lung nodules are detected quite commonly on CT scans of the chest. Half of the smokers who are 50 years and older have pulmonary nodules on CT examinations. Although the incidence of carcinoma in nodules in the 8-mm range is approximately 10% to 20%, the incidence of nodules smaller than 4 mm is less than 1%.[13] Overall, more than 90% of pulmonary nodules discovered serendipitously on CT chest scans are ultimately shown to be benign.[14] Data from a pilot study for the National Lung Screening Trial showed a cumulative incidence of 33% of false-positive results after 2 CT examinations; 7% of these patients required invasive testing to determine that the screening-detected lesion was not cancer.[15] Clearly most noncalcified pulmonary nodules can be classified as clinically insignificant incidentalomas.

Berland[12] has pointed out that there are many other incidentalomas. Some may be of little clinical relevance but nonetheless have potential clinical consequences, such as hiatal hernias, gallstones, splenomegaly, and renal calculi; others have no clinical importance such as renal or hepatic cysts and calcified granulomas of the liver or spleen.

THE DOWNSIDE OF REPORTING INCIDENTALOMAS: OVERDIAGNOSIS

The dilemma of whether to report all incidentalomas is not to be ignored. Radiologists neither want to get sued nor want to harm patients,[16] but the fact is that both options are quite real. In the unlikely event that an incidentaloma thought to be an entirely clinically insignificant finding should later have been found to have been an early carcinoma, the radiologist who failed to report the incidentaloma may well to be sued for malpractice and, as has been shown earlier, could well be found liable by a jury.

Reporting clinically insignificant incidentalomas can, on the other hand, result in overdiagnosis, a term used when a condition is diagnosed that would otherwise not go on to cause symptoms or death.[17] A classic example of this is illustrated by the experience of Casarella,[18] former Chairman of the Department of Radiology of Emory

University School of Medicine. Casarella underwent a CT colonography as part of a routine annual physical examination. His colon was reported as normal, but a renal lesion, a hepatic mass, and multiple noncalcified pulmonary nodules were discovered. A cascade of testing ensued. Contrast-enhanced CT scans of the abdomen demonstrated that the renal mass was simply a cyst, but the liver lesion was noncystic. CT scan of the lung revealed 8 small noncalcified nodules in the lung bases. CT-guided liver biopsy showed nonspecific granulomatous necrotic tissue. A positron emission tomography scan followed, which showed negative results. Thoracoscopy was then performed, during which 3 wedge resections of the right lung were taken. Pathologic diagnosis revealed noncalcified granulomas, probably related to old histoplasmosis.

But...there were complications. After the thoracoscopy, Casarella writes that he awoke in the recovery room with a "chest tube, a Foley catheter, a subclavian central venous catheter, a nasal oxygen catheter, an epidural catheter, an arterial catheter, subcutaneously administered heparin, a constant infusion of prophylactic antibiotics, and patient-controlled analgesia with intravenously administered narcotics." He made a slow recovery and even after being discharged home, pain and discomfort lingered but eventually resolved. In the final analysis, no significant disease was found, but Casarella had undergone extensive invasive testing with the considerable disabling pain and discomfort. Total hospital charges exceeded $50000. Casarella[18] concluded

> Routine screening...with CT will produce more [incidentalomas and] surgery and certainly more CT scans to monitor change. We as radiologists must understand the consequences to the patient. It is not nihilistic to suggest that more research is needed, and we need to prove that searching for occult lesions will improve the length and the quality of life.

Insofar as cancer overdiagnosis is concerned, the term is used either when the cancer never progresses or, in fact, actually regresses or when the cancer progresses slowly enough that the patient dies from other causes before the cancer becomes symptomatic. In a carefully detailed and extensively researched article, researchers Welch and Black[17] conclude that overdiagnosis occurs in 25% of mammographically detected breast cancers, 50% of chest radiography–detected lung cancers, 60% of prostate-specific antigen–detected prostate cancers, and a significant percentage of cases of neuroblastoma,

thyroid cancer, melanoma, and kidney cancer. In an accompanying editorial, the University of California, San Francisco (UCSF) researchers Esserman and Thompson[19] asked rhetorically, "Is it too risky to not biopsy and to potentially miss a cancer?" They answered

> Perhaps it is just the opposite. It is too risky to continue on the path where we are compelled to know what every lesion is, and then invoking the occulopathologic reflex, the reflexive need to treat anything that resembles cancer. We need to curb the urge to intervene with more thought and about what is truly valuable. We can ill afford to spend resources for diagnosis and treatment if we do not make a material contribution to a person's well-being.

In a similar commentary, MD Anderson Cancer Center radiologist Ginsberg[20] wrote

> Should it be the radiologist's obligation to track down every last potential abnormality, or is there a point where minor or likely irrelevant observations should be underplayed so as to prevent the overuse of imaging technology? I would argue that no; we are not obliged to mention every irrelevant finding.... [Unfortunately], some radiologists who are justifiable leery of liability claims feel compelled to mention minor findings that more confident or less fearful radiologists might ignore or soft pedal.

Berland[21] has echoed similar sentiments, pointing out that many radiologists feel that, "Uncertainty about small or indeterminate findings should be reduced to nearly zero; but failing to do so is one of the greatest risks for liability."

Other researchers have simply portrayed the dilemma of overdiagnosis as a question, "What is responsible use of information that nobody asked for but once found is difficult to ignore?"[22] The dilemma remains without definitive resolution.

WHAT SHOULD WE TELL PATIENTS

University of Rochester Medical Center researchers recently observed that a patient's right-to autonomy must be balanced with the ethical obligations of physicians to do good for patients (beneficence) and to not harm them (nonmaleficence).[23] The researchers go on to contend that, "more information is not always better. Dumping all available information on patients can be overwhelming and may paradoxically undermine their ability to choose wisely."

They conclude that "clinicians should withhold information that is likely to overwhelm and distress patients if their having the information will provide no obvious benefit and they don't ask for it."

Notwithstanding the perspective stated earlier, withholding information from patients presents many obstacles. Patients want to be informed of any abnormalities found in their radiological examinations or other tests. Indeed, one survey disclosed that 92% of patients wanted to be given results of their examinations directly from radiologists, whether those results were normal or abnormal.[24] In an autobiography written by Jordan,[25] who was Chief of Staff during the administration of President Jimmy Carter and who had suffered from multiple malignancies during his life, it was pointed out that, "Waiting for doctors to read your x-rays must be like waiting for the jury foreman in a capital punishment trial to read your verdict. All it takes is a little spot on the x-ray to indicate that you have cancer." Kolata,[26] medical reporter for the New York Times, several years ago wrote a front page article entitled "Sick, Scared, and Waiting." Kolata highlighted the enormous degree of anxiety experienced by a woman with a history of breast cancer who had undergone a CT scan to evaluate a lung lesion, "She waited by the phone for two days with a racing pulse, dry mouth, total preoccupation with what-ifs to the point that real life doesn't exist, willing the phone to ring. The woman didn't let anyone else use the phone. Her doctor never called, and the patient never spoke to him again." Patients undergoing radiological studies are worried and fearful about the results of these studies. If an abnormality or even a questionable abnormality is discovered and they are not told about it, the worry and fear often is transformed to hostility and anger, which often leads to litigation.

However, on the other side of the coin, patients may resent being told too much. Another New York Times reporter, Angier,[27,28] wrote about her own experience. She underwent a routine prenatal sonogram and was told by the physician that her baby appeared to have a club foot anomaly. She prepared for the worst but later gave birth to a normal baby. Under a headline entitled, "Ultrasound and Fury: One Mother's Ordeal," Angier lashed out at the ultrasonography physician because she was not fully informed about how imperfect ultrasonography is, how many false-positives that can have devastating outcomes occur, and the degree of uncertainty about ultrasound findings. "Women should be told that ultrasound is a serious procedure designed to look for abnormalities, but there are no guarantees," she concluded.[27,28]

A decade ago, the UCSF radiologist Filly[29] wrote an editorial dealing with his duty to inform patients of questionable abnormalities found on their prenatal ultrasound scans. He pointed out that often sonograms contain abnormalities such as a choroid plexus cyst, echogenic intracardiac foci, mild pyelectasis, or echogenic bowel, which may or may not be real abnormalities. The radiologist went on to write that Down syndrome markers of echogenic intracardiac foci occur in close to 10% of normal fetuses, choroid plexus cysts in 1% to 2%, echogenic bowel in more than 10%, and mild pyelectasis in 3%. Filly then asked rhetorically what the radiologist performing a routine sonogram who finds one of these markers of disease should tell the mother-to-be. This was his response:

If you have a busy sonographic practice seeing 10 to 20 pregnant women daily, you will likely see at least one of these "abnormalities" every day. Physicians in the trenches…identify these "abnormalities" during a routine sonogram. What are they to tell the patient? Once the parents are informed of this "abnormality," enjoyment of the anticipation of the birth of their son or daughter is now replaced by anxiety.

From my vantage point, the identification of these "abnormalities" in low-risk women has crossed the line of "more harm than good"-….Think about it! For the tiny residual number of Down syndrome fetuses that may potentially come to light by chasing down every last marker," we intend to put at least 10% of all pregnant women with a perfectly normal fetus through a great deal of worry.

So then what should I do tomorrow? Should I have the courage of my conviction to simply ignore these features? I wish I had that courage, but I don't. Even with my considerable clout in the world of obstetric sonography, I cannot unilaterally ignore the sonographic medical literature. That is not how American medicine works.

In her novel entitled Handle with Care, novelist Picoult[30] focused on a woman who gave birth to a child with osteogenesis imperfecta. The new mother later discovered that the obstetrician who had performed the prenatal ultrasonography had in fact suspected the possibility of the presence of osteogenesis imperfecta, but had not said anything about the finding to the mother-to-be. The mother later filed a wrongful birth medical malpractice lawsuit alleging that the obstetrician's failure to have informed her of the possibility that her baby night have osteogenesis imperfecta prevented her from electing to have an abortion. At the ensuing trial, the plaintiff's attorney said to the jury

This case is about facts—facts that the obstetrician knew and dismissed. Facts that weren't given to a patient by a physician she trusted. No one is blaming the obstetrician for the child's condition; no one is saying the obstetrician caused the illness. However, the obstetrician is to blame for not giving the family all the information that was available…. When a physician withholds information from a patient, that's malpractice.

The Code of Ethics of the American Medical Association states "The physician's obligation is to present the medical facts accurately to the patient…. Physicians should disclose all relevant medical information to patients."[31] The dilemma about what, if anything, physicians should inform patients of incidentalomas, particularly those that may or may not be an early cancer, is realistically illustrated by a *New York Times* editorial[32]:

The ability of screening tests to detect very tiny tumors has outstripped our understanding of how to interpret and respond to the findings. For decades it has been an article of faith that early detection is a surefire way to save lives. It seems intuitively obvious that detecting a tumor very early will result in the best chance for cure. But this has been challenged recently. A key issue is whether the tests are findings tumors that would never become dangerous but cannot be distinguished from tumors that could become deadly, causing many patients to undergo unnecessary risks of surgery, radiation, and chemotherapy.

In courtroom trials, juries decide whether or not the defendant is liable for malpractice. Juries are composed of jurors who are members of the public. About 87% of surveyed adults believe that routine cancer screening is almost always a good idea and that finding cancer saves lives early,[33] and 68% of women believe that screening prevents or reduces the risk of contracting breast cancer.[34] Even the fact that 43% of persons undergoing screening tests experience at least 1 false-positive result does not seem to limit the public's almost insatiable demand for continued testing.[35] Another survey disclosed that 75% eligible jurors said that they would act on their own beliefs, regardless of legal instructions from the judge.[36] Thus, even if the likelihood that a particular incidentaloma represents a serious disease such as cancer is extremely small, that is if the incidentaloma does indeed turn out to be a serious disease, convincing a jury that a defendant radiologist who withheld from the patient the existence of that incidentaloma is not liable for malpractice seems to be most difficult.

CONNECTION BETWEEN OVEREXPOSURE TO IMAGING USING IONIZING RADIATION AND CANCER

Although this article has focused predominantly on the medical malpractice risks associated with failing to identify and report incidentalomas that may later develop into cancers or other serious disease and the risks associated with complications that may arise from the unnecessary cascade of tests that are performed because of overemphasizing apparently insignificant incidentalomas, some mention ought to be made about the risks of radiation exposure. Exposure to imaging involving radiation and the hazards related to such exposure have myriad medical-legal ramifications. Data regarding increasing exposure to ionizing radiation emanating from radiological procedures are startling. Americans were exposed to more than 7 times as much ionizing radiation from diagnostic medical procedures in 2006 than they were in the early 1980s.[37] Although in 1980, medical imaging was responsible for only 15% of the total radiation exposure to the population in the United States, now the proportion has risen to 50%.[38] This rate of exposure is alarming to much of the public at large because some researchers have estimated that eventually 29000 cancers every year, half of which would be fatal, could be the result of past CT scan use.[39] A *USA Today* headline proclaimed that, "Overuse of diagnostic CT scans may cause 3 million excess cancers in the united states over the next 2–3 decades."[40] A recent editorial in the *Archives of Internal Medicine* stated, "What is becoming clear is that the large doses of radiation from the 19500 CT scans performed every day in the United States will translate, statistically, into additional cancers."[41]

Can radiologists' recommending CT scans and other imaging studies using ionizing radiation for incidentalomas that have an extremely low likelihood of representing serious disease lead to development of cancer in a patient who in turn may file a medical malpractice lawsuit against the interpreting radiologist? At present, clearly there is insufficient data available from the scientific community to justify an unequivocal determination of whether cancer can or cannot develop from diagnostic-level radiation used in radiological imaging. Thus far, there have never been successful medical malpractice lawsuits that allege development of cancer or genetic defects resulting from diagnostic radiographic examinations. However, courts are open to any aggrieved individual who wishes to file a lawsuit, and in civil litigation, judges and juries decide matters based not on certainty but rather on the basis of "more likely than not" (ie, more than 50%). The courts are unlikely to ever decide with certainty whether diagnostic-level radiation is carcinogenic, but on a case-by-case basis, they will not shirk from deciding whether a liability is imposed when such allegations are made. It is quite likely that lawsuits alleging development of cancer arising from diagnostic imaging using current levels of ionizing radiation will be forthcoming. How the courts will deal with these issues remains to be determined.

SUMMARY

Serendipitous discovery by radiologists on radiographic examinations of findings unrelated to the reason for which the radiographic examination was ordered in the first place, that is, incidental findings, is certainly nothing new. However, with the advent of CT and its properties of high resolution and extremely thin cross-sectional images, radiologists began to observe body structures and organ variations that had been virtually invisible on standard radiography. Magnetic resonance imaging and ultrasonography expanded this ability. Although most of these newly visible findings are easily identified as either definite normal structure variations or definite pathologic lesions, many of the findings not related to the reason for the examination that are incidentally found are indeterminant. These findings are incidentalomas. As imaging technology advances, the frequency of incidentalomas increases proportionately.

Incidentalomas identified on radiological studies present a dilemma for radiologists. If the radiologist believes beyond reasonable doubt that a given incidentaloma is of no clinical significance, then making mention of it in his radiological report may well lead to a cascade of tests, sometimes resulting in biopsies or other surgical procedures. And on occasion a biopsy or surgical procedure performed for an incidentaloma of no clinical significance can lead to serious complications. On the other hand, if the radiologist decides to not mention the incidentaloma in the radiological report and in the unlikely event the incidentaloma later turns out to have been an early carcinoma or finding of other significant disease, then the patient's health has been severely jeopardized and medical malpractice litigation could well ensue.

Although this article focuses on radiological imaging, it should be noted that the dilemma of managing incidentalomas is certainly not limited to radiologists. Recent articles point out that incidentalomas present similar dilemmas for researchers working in genomic medicine,[42,43] newborn screening,[44] and neuroimaging.[45]

The question of whether to report or not report incidentalomas is not easily answered. It is likely that specific situations in which radiologists over-call or undercall incidentalomas will generate occasional medical malpractice lawsuits. How judges and juries will resolve such lawsuits cannot be predicted.

REFERENCES

1. Brant WE, Helms CA. Fundamentals of diagnostic radiology. Baltimore (MD): Williams & Wilkins; 1994. p. 483.
2. Juhl JH, Crummy AB, Kuhlman JE. Essentials of radiologic imaging. Philadelphia: Lippincott-Raven; 1998. p. 787.
3. Schloendorff v The Society of New York Hosp, 105 NE 92 (NY 1914).
4. Duckworth v Lutheran Med Ctr 1995 WL 33070, (OH App.1995).
5. Berlin L. Failure to diagnose lung cancer: anatomy of a malpractice trial. AJR Am J Roentgenol 2003;180: 37–45.
6. Werth B. Damages. New York: Simon & Schuster; 1998. p. 54.
7. Berlin L. Hindsight bias. AJR Am J Roentgenol 2000; 175:597–601.
8. Berlin L. Outcome bias. AJR Am J Roentgenol 2004; 183:557–60.
9. Cronan JJ. Thyroid nodules: is it time to turn off the US machines? Radiology 2008;247:602–4.
10. Shirodkar M, Jabbour SA. Endocrine incidentalomas. Int J Clin Pract 2008;62:1423–31.
11. Song JH, Chaudhry FS, Mayo-Smith WW. The incidental adrenal mass on CT: prevalence of adrenal disease in 1049 consecutive adrenal masses in patients with no known malignancy. AJR Am J Roentgenol 2008;190:1163–8.
12. Berland LL. Incidental extracolonic findings on CT colonography: the impending deluge and its implications. J Am Coll Radiol 2009;6:14–20.
13. MacMahon H, Austin JHM, Gamsu G, et al. Guidelines for management of small pulmonary nodules detected on CT scans: a statement from the Fleischner Society. Radiology 2005;237:395–400.
14. Ravenel JG, Costello P, Silvestri GA. Screening for lung cancer. AJR Am J Roentgenol 2008;190:755–61.
15. Croswell JM, Baker SG, Marcus PM, et al. Cumulative incidence of false-positive test results in lung

cancer screening: a randomized trial. Ann Intern Med 2010;152:505–12.

16. Warshauer DM. The age of (over) discovery. J Am Coll Radiol 2010;7:246–7.

17. Welch HG, Black WC. Overdiagnosis in cancer. J Natl Cancer Inst 2010;102:605–13.

18. Casarella WJ. A patient's viewpoint on a current controversy. Radiology 2002;224:927.

19. Esserman L, Thompson I. Solving the overdiagnosis dilemma. J Natl Cancer Inst 2010;102:582–3.

20. Ginsberg LE. "If clinically indicated:" is it? Radiology 2010;254:324–5.

21. Berland LL. Incidentalomas on CT colonography: do not make a mountain out of a molehill [author's reply]. J Am Coll Radiol 2009;6:599–600.

22. Fletcher RH, Pignone M. Extracolonic findings with computed tomographic colonography: asset or liability? Arch Intern Med 2008;168:685–6.

23. Epstein RM, Korones DN, Quill TE. Withholding information from patients: when less is more. N Engl J Med 2010;362:380–1.

24. Schreiber MH, Leonard M, Rieniets CY. Disclosure of imaging findings to patients directly by radiologists: survey of patients' preferences. AJR Am J Roentgenol 1995;165:467–9.

25. Jordan H. No such thing as a bad day. Atlanta (GA): Longstreet Press; 2000. p. 153.

26. Kolata G. Sick and scared, and waiting, waiting, waiting. New York Times August 20, 2005;A1.

27. Angier N. Ultrasound and fury: one mother's ordeal. New York Times November 26, 1996. Available at: http://www.nytimes.com/1996/11/26/science/ultrasound-and-fury-one-mother-s-ordeal.html. Accessed May 24, 2010.

28. Angier N. Doctors favor ultrasound use in right hands. New York Times July 15, 1997. Available at: http://www.nytimes.com/1997/07/15/science/doctors-favor-ultrasound-use-in-right-hands.html. Accessed May 24, 2010.

29. Filly RA. Obstetrical sonography: the best way to terrify a pregnant woman [editorial]. J Ultrasound Med 2000;19:1–5.

30. Picoult J. Handle with care. New York: Simon & Schuster; 2009. p. 337.

31. American Medical Association Council on ethical and judicial affairs. Code of medical ethics 2008–2009 Edition; 8. 08, Informed Consent 2008:245–6.

32. Cancer screening and the individual [editorial]. New York Times April 14, 2002;A12.

33. Schwartz LM, Woloshin S, Fowler FJ, et al. Enthusiasm for cancer screening in the United States. JAMA 2004;291:71–8.

34. Domenighetti G, D'Avanzo B, Egger M, et al. Women's perception of the benefits of mammography screening: population-based survey in four countries. Int J Epidemiol 2003;32:816–21.

35. Lafata JE, Simpkins J, Lamerato L, et al. The economic impact of false-positive cancer screens. Cancer Epidemiol Biomarkers Prev 2004;13:2116–32.

36. Lester W. Jurors say they follow beliefs, not instructions. Chicago Sun Times October 24, 1998;37.

37. Schauer DA, Linton OW. National council on radiation protection and measurements report shows substantial medical exposure increase. Radiology 2009;253:293–6.

38. Brenner DJ. Medical imaging in the 21st century: getting the best bang for the rad. N Engl J Med 2010;362:943–5.

39. deGonzalez AB, Mahadevappa M, Kim KP, et al. Projected cancer risks from computed tomographic scans performed in the United States in 2007. Arch Intern Med 2009;169:2071–7.

40. Sternberg S. Unnecessary CT scans exposing patients to excessive radiation. USA Today November 29, 2007;A1.

41. Redberg RF. Cancer risks and radiation exposure from computed tomographic scans: how can we be sure the benefits outweigh the risks? Arch Intern Med 2009;169:2049–50.

42. Kohane IS, Masys DR, Altman RB. The incidentaloma: a threat to genomic medicine. JAMA 2006; 296:212–5.

43. Wolf SM, Kahn JP, Nelson CA. The incidentaloma [letters]. JAMA 2006;296:2800–1.

44. Tarini BA. The current revolution in newborn screening: new technology, old controversies. Arch Pediatr Adolesc Med 2007;161(8):767–72.

45. Rangel EK. The management of incidental findings in neuro-imaging research: framework and recommendations. J Law Med Ethics 2010;38(1): 117–26.

The Economic Burden of Incidentally Detected Findings

Alexander Ding, MD, MS[a], Jonathan D. Eisenberg, BA[b],
Pari V. Pandharipande, MD, MPH[b,c],*

KEYWORDS

• Economic burden • Incidental findings • Imaging
• CT colonography

Practitioners in all medical disciplines recognize the high frequency of incidentally detected findings, that is, findings that do not have associated clinical symptoms. Although some findings are discovered on physical examination, an increasing majority are detected at imaging performed for another indication. In addition to their medical implications, incidental findings can be associated with substantial downstream costs.[1–16] The economic burden of these findings, however, has been sparsely studied in the published literature to date. With increasing federal scrutiny on the net value of imaging services, the costs and benefits of incidental findings need to be more rigorously quantified. In this article, the authors examine current related work and provide a framework for future investigations that will efficiently and substantially advance the knowledge in this field.

Because of unprecedented advances in imaging technology in recent years, there has been a remarkable increase in the demand for imaging. From 1995 to 2005, the number of computed tomographic (CT) scans obtained for Medicare beneficiaries more than doubled and the number of magnetic resonance (MR) imaging scans more than tripled,[17] a trend substantiated in the private sector as well.[18] As practitioners increasingly rely on cross-sectional imaging, they are faced with an increasing burden of incidental findings. In a retrospectively identified contemporary cohort of patients who underwent 1426 imaging studies in the setting of clinical research, 567 (39.8%) had a minimum of 1 incidental finding.[19] Further work up definitively benefited patients in 6 cases (1.1%) in which significant infections or neoplasms were identified.[19] Although incidental findings occasionally present an opportunity to cure or halt an otherwise lethal disease, many downstream consequences are unfavorable. For patients, these findings can create anxiety and additional work up for findings that are ultimately benign or unlikely to affect their life expectancy. For busy practitioners, the recommended follow-up can be difficult to organize and can detract care from more important medical issues. Furthermore, these consequences can translate into substantial downstream expenditures.

In this era of national federally mandated health care reform, when making reimbursement decisions about imaging in a variety of health care paradigms, policymakers will want to know not only the true costs of incidental findings but, more specifically, how such costs affect the net value of a given imaging strategy. Moving forward, investigators should consider incidental findings explicitly when evaluating the value or cost-effectiveness of an imaging strategy. This approach is important because a high frequency of incidental findings (and associated expenditures) may be acceptable,

a Department of Radiology, Massachusetts General Hospital, 55 Fruit Street, Boston, MA 02114, USA
b Department of Radiology, Institute for Technology Assessment, Massachusetts General Hospital, 101 Merrimac Street, 10th floor, Boston, MA 02114, USA
c Department of Radiology, Harvard Medical School, Boston, MA, USA
* Corresponding author. Department of Radiology, Institute for Technology Assessment, Massachusetts General Hospital, 101 Merrimac Street, 10th floor, Boston, MA 02114.
E-mail address: pari@mgh-ita.org

Radiol Clin N Am 49 (2011) 257–265
doi:10.1016/j.rcl.2010.11.004

for example, in a situation in which an imaging study appropriately and uniquely detects a disease. In contrast, an imaging study that already has marginal value for detecting a given disease may be of even lesser value if a disproportionate number of incidental findings are detected.

At this point in time, much work remains to be done in this field. Some relevant studies have investigated the short-term costs associated with incidental findings at imaging, particularly when performed in a screening context.[1–16] However, estimates of comprehensive, long-term, societal costs consequent to imaging-detected incidental findings are largely absent. Furthermore, there is not yet a consistent precedent, within the imaging literature, for estimating the long-term health and economic outcomes of incidental findings along-side primary long-term outcomes that are relevant to original study indications. In this review, the authors: (1) provide an overview of the existing literature on imaging-detected incidental findings and their economic burden, focusing on 3 examination types, abdominal/pelvic CT, chest CT, and cardiac CT, which have been the subject of most relevant studies to date[1–16] and (2) provide insight as to how to fill critical research gaps to better quantify the true economic burden of imaging-detected incidental findings in the health care system.

ABDOMINAL IMAGING
CT Colonography

Concerns about the economic impact of incidental extracolonic findings at CT colonography (CTC) have had a greater impact at the policy level than any other context of incidental findings.[20–22] Although robust data that quantify the long-term costs of extracolonic findings are not yet available, concerns about the magnitude of this burden have contributed to skepticism among policymakers about the net value of CTC for population-level screening.[21,22] Of particular importance, these concerns weighed into the decision of the Centers for Medicare and Medicaid Services in 2009 to decline reimbursement for CTC.[23] In this section, the authors provide an overview of published data on the costs of extracolonic findings, including studies done within and outside of the United States.[1–10] Of note, from an economic perspective, these reported costs are considered to be short term in horizon; the longest reported mean follow-up period among studies was 3.6 years.[10] The authors also examine the potential benefits of a proposed classification system for extracolonic CTC findings for improving future efforts to quantify the economic burden of extracolonic findings.[2,4,24]

Several US studies have investigated the scope of incidental findings detected at CTC and the associated short-term costs of these findings.[2–7,10] Cumulatively, in 7 primary series, incidental findings were reported in 41% to 98% of cases, of which the findings were clinically significant in 7% to 18% of cases, resulting in added work up costs of $13 to $248 per scan (Table 1).[2–7,10] Importantly, these studies varied significantly in the types of costs included. Of the 7 studies, 5 reported only added costs due to medical imaging or other diagnostic tests.[2–5,10] Hara and colleagues,[5] in a prospective study of 264 patients, found that 30 of 264 (11.4%) scans had clinically significant extracolonic findings, generating a mean additional cost of $28 per scan over the entire screening cohort. Gluecker and colleagues[3] confirmed the results in a larger cohort from the same institution, finding additional costs of $34 per patient screened. Yee and colleagues[10] subsequently published their results in a large prospectively followed screening cohort and found that extracolonic findings resulted in additional work up costs of $28 per patient screened. Flicker and colleagues[2] and Veerappan and colleagues[4] reported added costs due to imaging alone[2] and imaging plus other diagnostic tests[4]; these 2 studies are discussed in greater detail later in the context of a classification system for extracolonic findings.[24]

Two studies instead reported total work up costs, including treatment.[6,7] Pickhardt and colleagues,[7] in a retrospective study of 2195 patients, found that clinically significant extracolonic findings were detected in 157 (7.2%) CTC scans. Relevant new diagnoses were made in 2.5% of patients, including 9 previously unknown malignancies.[7] For the work up of extracolonic findings, the mean cost per patient screened was $99, with $31 attributed to nonsurgical costs (including further imaging) and $68 attributed to surgical and inpatient hospital costs.[7] In 136 asymptomatic patients, Kimberly and colleagues[6] found that 134 (98.5%) had at least 1 extracolonic finding and that 25 (17.5%) patients had clinically significant extracolonic findings. The average cost for evaluating the extracolonic findings was $248 per patient screened, $185 for additional imaging, $8 for laboratory studies, $38 for procedures, and $17 for outpatient visits.[6] The investigators noted that their higher reported costs, relative to prior studies, may have been because of their practice of reporting all extracolonic findings to primary care physicians without further specific guidance regarding work up.[6]

Analogous studies from the United Kingdom[8,9] and Australia[1] have yielded comparable results (see Table 1). In a prospective Australian study

Table 1
CT colonography studies reporting added costs of incidental findings

Authors	Journal	Year	Location	Study Type	Population	Cohort Mean Age (y)	Number of Cases	Incidental Findings Percentage (%)	Clinically Significant Percentage (%)	Average Added Cost Per Scan ($)
Hara et al[5]	Radiology	2000	United States	Prospective	Asymptomatic	64	264	41	11	28[c]
Gluecker et al[3]	Gastroenterology	2003	United States	Prospective	Asymptomatic	64[a]	681	69	10	34[c]
Yee et al[10]	Radiology	2005	United States	Prospective	Mixed	63	500	63	9	28[c]
Chin et al[1]	Am J Gastroenterol	2005	Australia	Prospective	Asymptomatic	59	432	27	7	24[d]
Xiong et al[9]	Br J Radiol	2006	United Kingdom	Prospective	Symptomatic	74[a]	225	52	N/A	282[b,e]
Tolan et al[8]	AJR	2007	United Kingdom	Retrospective	Symptomatic	80	400	67	29	67[d]
Flicker et al[2]	JCAT	2008	United States	Retrospective	Mixed	61	376	72	18	13[c]
Pickhardt et al[7]	Radiology	2008	United States	Retrospective	Asymptomatic	58	2195	N/A	7	99[e]
Kimberly et al[6]	J Gen Intern Med	2008	United States	Prospective	Mixed	57[a]	136	98	18	248[e]
Veerappan et al[4]	AJR	2010	United States	Retrospective	Asymptomatic	59	2277	46	11	50[d]

Abbreviation: N/A, not specifically addressed.
[a] Median reported instead of mean.
[b] Converted based on 2006 rates.[25]
[c] Includes imaging-related costs.
[d] Includes imaging-related and other diagnostic costs.
[e] Includes imaging-related costs as well as other diagnostic and treatment costs.

of 432 asymptomatic patients, 146 (27.3%) patients had extracolonic findings, of which 32 (7.4%) were deemed clinically significant.[1] Added work up costs of clinic visits, further imaging, and laboratory tests amounted to an extra $24 per scan when averaged over the entire cohort.[1] In a prospective study of 225 symptomatic patients in the United Kingdom, 116 (51.6%) CTC scans performed had extracolonic findings; 24 (10.7%) generated further work up.[9] Additional costs generated by CTC were £153 (US $282)[25] per scan when averaged over the entire cohort, most of which were from surgical procedures.[9] In a retrospective UK study of 400 symptomatic patients, 268 (67%) scans performed were associated with extracolonic findings; 116 (29%) scans had clinically significant findings.[8] Among this population, 45 patients underwent further work up and 22 were diagnosed with new extracolonic malignancies.[8] The total cost of work up for extracolonic findings was £34 (US $67) per scan when averaged over the entire cohort.[8]

An important limitation to consider when comparing the costs of extracolonic CTC findings across investigations is the wide variation in the classification of these findings. This variability is substantiated by a wide reported range in the prevalence of extracolonic findings (41%–98%) (see **Table 1**).[1–3,5–10] To address this variability, Zalis and colleagues[24] developed a classification system for extracolonic findings, with the goal of improving both clinical care and research relevant to CTC findings. Flicker and colleagues[2] subsequently reported their findings when applying this classification system to a retrospective group of 376 patients who underwent CTC. The investigators found that 272 (72.3%) scans had extracolonic findings; 51 (13.6%) had E3 findings (likely unimportant but incompletely characterized and work up may be indicated) and 16 (4.3%) had E4 findings (potentially important and should be communicated to the referring physician).[2] The extra cost of working up these lesions amounted to $13 per screening scan when averaged over the entire cohort.[2] Veerappan and colleagues[4] also applied the classification system to a retrospectively identified screening cohort. In their study of 2277 patients, they reported extracolonic findings in 1037 patients (45.5%), including 211 (9.3%) patients with E3 findings and 39 (1.7%) with E4 findings.[4] Costs resulting from the work up of these findings totaled $50 per patient, when averaged over the entire cohort.[4] This system, if universally adopted, could help to ensure that referrals for the evaluation of extracolonic lesions are done more consistently. Ultimately, consistent reporting is critical for understanding the true economic burden of incidental extracolonic findings at CTC. As noted earlier, the magnitude of this burden may substantially influence the viability of CTC for colorectal cancer screening in the future.

Abdominal CT–Non-CTC Indications

Although CTC represents a setting in which the economic burden of incidental findings is of foremost concern from a policy perspective, abdominal CT performed for other indications accounts for most incidental findings in abdominal imaging.[11,12,26] However, as in the case of CTC, published data informing attendant costs are limited. In a prospective study of 344 patients undergoing CT urography for the evaluation of hematuria, Liu and colleagues[11] found that 259 (75.3%) had extraurinary incidental findings; 62 (18.0%) had incidental findings deemed of high clinical significance. Among the 344 patients, 8.4% underwent further diagnostic imaging at an added cost of $41 when averaged over all scans initially performed.[11] In a retrospective study of 175 CT angiography (CTA) studies performed on renal donor candidates, Maizlin and colleagues[12] reported 71 (40.6%) patients to have extrarenal incidental findings; 18 (10.3%) had findings of high clinical significance. The further recommended follow-up studies added an estimated $35 per scan, when averaged over all scans performed.[12] Further research is needed to better understand the economic burden of incidental findings across the wide spectrum of common clinical indications for abdominal CT.

THORACIC IMAGING

Among chest CT indications, lung cancer screening, if widely adopted for high-risk patients such as smokers, may generate the highest burden of incidental findings.[14,27] While incidental findings, detection of nonmalignant nodules, and competing risks of mortality are all expected to influence the cost-effectiveness of lung cancer screening in smokers, a comprehensive cost-effectiveness analysis has not yet been reported.[14,27–29] Investigators have attempted to quantify the magnitude of incidental findings at screening chest CT and their short-term costs. MacRedmond and colleagues[27] reported a prevalence of 62% of incidental findings at screening chest CT, most commonly emphysema and coronary artery disease. In a retrospective Canadian study of 4073 patients who received screening chest CT scans, Kucharczyk and colleagues[14] found that 782 (19.2%) patients had incidental findings; 486 (11.9%) patients required imaging follow-up. Ultimately, 7 biopsy-proven cancers were diagnosed, 4 breast cancers, 2 rib plasmacytomas, and 1 thyroid cancer.[14] Per screening chest CT examination performed, the added costs of further diagnostic work up were estimated to be Can$12.[14] Of specific note, these studies did not include lung nodules as incidental findings; although a large percentage of detected lung nodules are benign at CT, their detection and work up is related to the clinical indication of lung cancer screening, and thus they are not considered incidental. In the setting of most other chest CT indications, for example, cardiac CT, as discussed later, incidental lung nodules contribute substantively to short- and long-term costs of incidental findings.

Importantly, thyroid abnormalities are also commonly incidentally detected at chest CT during imaging of the lower neck. More than 50% of asymptomatic patients have thyroid nodules at autopsy[30]; therefore, the likelihood of encountering a thyroid nodule on a CT or MR imaging study that includes a portion of the thyroid gland is high. Yousem and colleagues[13] retrospectively analyzed 231 CT and MR imaging studies of the neck and found 36 (15.6%) to demonstrate incidental thyroid nodules. Of all cases, 2.6% underwent further work up. The cost of further work up and treatment was $31 when averaged over all patients scanned.[13]

CARDIAC IMAGING

A well-known debate about cardiac CT is whether or not to limit the field-of-view to the heart, an issue driven largely by the burden of extracardiac incidental findings. Many argue that a major salient limitation of cardiac CT is the high rate of pulmonary nodule detection and the extent to which this causes low yield, unanticipated follow-up and interventions, as well as increased costs.[16]

Early investigations have begun to quantify the extent of extracardiac incidental findings and their attendant short-term costs. A literature review by Sosnouski and colleagues[31] noted that incidental extracardiac findings were present on coronary CTA in 25% to 61% of studies. Lee and colleagues[16] retrospectively studied 151 patients who underwent full-field cardiac CT and found that 65 (43.0%) patients had incidental findings; in 47 patients (31.1%), findings were deemed potentially clinically significant. Despite recommendations for work up for 19 findings, only 6 patients received further work up, 1 in whom a malignancy was detected and treated.[16] Of note, a high prevalence of incidental pulmonary nodules was observed, 55% of patients (26/47) with potentially significant incidental findings had

pulmonary nodules larger than 4 mm.[16] The direct costs of additional work up were $17.42 per patient, when averaged over the entire cohort studied.[16] Machaalany and colleagues[15] prospectively studied 966 Canadian patients evaluated with full-field-of-view cardiac CT and found that 401 (41.5%) patients showed extracardiac findings. These findings were classified into clinically significant (12/966, 1.2%), indeterminate (68/966, 7.0%), and clinically nonsignificant (321/966, 33.2%) categories.[15] A total of 164 additional imaging studies and procedures were performed for the 80 patients with clinically significant or indeterminate findings; 6 patients were ultimately diagnosed and treated for malignancy.[15] Direct costs of investigating all incidental findings were Can$60 (US $86) per scanned patient.[15]

PRIMARY LIMITATIONS OF ECONOMIC INVESTIGATIONS TO DATE

To date, most published literature on the economic burden of incidental findings is centered on CT of the chest and abdomen in adults.[1–3,5–16] Cost analyses of incidental findings seen during neurologic, musculoskeletal, or pediatric imaging are sparse or absent. In addition, most studies address screening scenarios. When performing imaging for symptoms or for a known disease process, the short-term costs of incidental findings may differ. For example, in a patient with a large hepatocellular carcinoma at CT, a questionable small renal lesion does not merit further work up in most cases because of the poor prognosis of the hepatic malignancy. However, in an asymptomatic patient without known comorbidities the renal finding may result in substantial further work up and attendant costs.

Furthermore, to date, reported added costs associated with incidental findings and their consequent work up have been modest, with most studies reporting added costs of less than $100 per scan performed.[1–16] However, these estimates may be artificially low. As noted, the types of costs included across investigations (eg, diagnostic work up costs, treatment costs) are variable.[1–16] A related limitation is that the time horizons of most analyses, the period from the detection of an incidental finding to the termination of patient follow-up and cost analysis, have been short and have not explicitly addressed life expectancy consequences (benefits or harms) of incidental findings.[1–16] These short follow-up periods constitute one of the largest limitations of this body of research. That being said, the resource requirements for tracking the long-term downstream costs and health consequences of incidental findings, particularly for large patient cohorts, are preclusive in many research settings.

To better understand the economic burden of incidental findings in imaging, there remains a significant amount of research to be done. Salient methods and issues to be investigated, particularly those that can efficiently and effectively advance this field, are discussed in detail below.

FUTURE RESEARCH DIRECTIONS
A Call for Economic Models

Economic models integrate multiple data sources, including costs, life expectancy, and quality of life (QOL), to predict the long-term downstream consequences and value of a given imaging test or procedure.[32–35] When considering methods for evaluating the economic burden of incidental findings, such models carry three primary advantages: (1) long-term downstream costs, benefits, and harms can be estimated, accounting for the costs of added procedures and complications as well as potential life expectancy gains or losses; (2) competing risks of morbidity and mortality, such as may be relevant with advanced age or concurrent disease processes, can be explicitly considered; and (3) a societal perspective can be achieved, making the results more generalizable than would be the case for a single-institution study.[35] Thus, economic models can provide a more realistic and comprehensive view of the economic burden of incidental findings than is typically possible through primary data collection. However, to develop robust economic models in this field, more primary data collection relevant to incidental findings is first needed. The authors describe what types of data are important to collect and how such data can be integrated to develop efficient models for economic analyses.

Classifying Incidental Findings During Primary Data Collection

To build robust economic models, more information is needed about the scope of incidental findings in each imaging subspecialty. Moreover, as investigators collect these data, there will be a critical need to classify these findings in a uniform fashion. Consider, for example, two investigative groups that are studying the same group of patients, all of whom received abdominal CT scans. One group may designate a renal cyst as an incidental finding, whereas the other group may not. If each group reports added costs per incidental finding, the results of their analyses will be different, even though they are studying the same group. A recently published consensus paper on the management of incidental findings

at abdominal CT generated by the American College of Radiology Incidental Findings Committttee[36] and the previously mentioned classification system for extracolonic findings proposed by Zalis and colleagues[24] for CTC represent important steps toward more uniform classification of incidental findings, but much more work is needed in this area.

Furthermore, the clinical and economic importance of most incidental findings depends on patient-specific factors. When investigators collect and classify data on incidental findings, patient-specific factors that could influence management decisions should be concurrently tracked and reported. Consider a small pancreatic cyst detected incidentally on an abdominal CT. The patient's age at detection influences the management of this finding, including follow-up imaging and cost requirements. This relationship between patient status and the burden of incidental findings merits specific consideration; investigators must be careful not to over- or underestimate the economic burden of incidental findings in one population by erroneously extrapolating cost data to another.

Addressing Cost Differences Related to Practice Heterogeneity

Estimating costs that are incurred as a consequence of incidental findings similarly requires a systematized transparent approach. The clinical course and outcomes of patients who have had incidental findings are defined by heterogeneous practitioner recommendations and patient adherence patterns; this spectrum of patient experience must be collected in detail. As described later, economic modeling techniques, in turn, allow this type of heterogeneity to be explicitly considered. For example, the economic impact of different levels of adherence to recommended follow-up imaging can be evaluated, ranging from 0% (no adherence) to 100% adherence. Heterogeneity in work up practices (eg, imaging-guided biopsy vs direct surgery for a solid incidental renal mass) can also be explicitly considered in a model to determine the economic consequences of different approaches.[34]

Developing Economic Models that Incorporate Incidental Findings

In economic analyses, when evaluating a diagnostic strategy for disease detection, long-term comprehensive costs are ideally estimated alongside consequent life expectancy; this method enables not just costs but the underlying value of the strategy to be estimated. Long-term cost and life expectancy projections can be concurrently estimated using a variety of biostatistical, Markov modeling, or Monte Carlo simulation techniques.[29,32,34,37] Importantly, these long-term projections are made not only for the diagnostic strategy under consideration but also for relevant alternative strategies. Recent relevant examples include cost-effectiveness analyses of CTC for colorectal cancer screening (relative to current standards, including optical colonoscopy),[32] MR imaging for breast cancer screening in *BRCA1* mutation carriers (relative to mammography),[33] and imaging-guided biopsy in patients with small renal masses (relative to empiric surgery).[34] Moving forward, incidental findings should ideally be incorporated within economic models that aim to evaluate the overall value of a given diagnostic imaging strategy. In this way, the attendant long-term costs and life expectancy implications of incidental findings can be integrated with other costs, risks, and benefits inherent to the imaging strategy under consideration for a given clinical indication. Thus, the impact of incidental findings on a strategy's underlying value can be evaluated explicitly.

Importantly, quality of life (QOL) is an integral component of economic analyses in medicine but has been sparsely studied to date in imaging practices.[38–41] The rationale for incorporating QOL into economic analyses in medicine and for adjusting life expectancy estimates to incorporate QOL (eg, quality-adjusted life years) is that to estimate how a society values health care services, the value that a society places on time spent in different states of health must be considered.[35] In the context of incidental findings, many argue that patient stress and inconvenience incurred during any additional recommended work up must be considered. However, equally important to consider is the anxiety that can result from forgoing the work up of a lesion with a low, but nonzero, likelihood of malignancy. These competing QOL forces merit further investigation. If practitioners only recommend further work up for incidental findings when they are highly likely to have clinical consequences, the economic burden of incidental findings could be reduced enormously. However, QOL influences must be considered when making related policy decisions to ensure that these decisions are well-aligned with societal preferences.

Cost-Effectiveness Analysis

When a model is developed to generate long-term cost and effectiveness data for competing health care strategies, a cost-effectiveness analysis can be performed to compare the relative value of the strategies under consideration.[35] Importantly, this type of analysis is structured to address a specific clinical scenario, for example, the cost-effectiveness of CTC relative to optical colonoscopy for colorectal cancer screening, and not a single diagnostic test in isolation. In a standard cost-effectiveness analysis, lifetime costs and quality-adjusted life expectancy are estimated for each diagnostic strategy under consideration and are simultaneously compared in an incremental cost-effectiveness analysis.[35] Within this type of analysis, as noted earlier, the extent to which incidental findings affect the cost and effectiveness of an imaging strategy under consideration can be explicitly evaluated. Importantly, this approach to estimating the economic burden of incidental findings is likely to yield more clinically meaningful results than isolated analyses of the costs of incidental findings because the former critically accounts for the original value of the imaging strategy under consideration for addressing the clinical question at hand.

SUMMARY

The use of medical imaging, particularly CT and MR imaging, has soared in the last several decades.[17,18] Over the same time period, the cost of medical care in the United States has been increasing at rates that are not economically sustainable. With increased scrutiny of the costs of medical care, imaging has been highlighted as an area of particular growth and cost.[18] Increased imaging use among practitioners results in an unavoidable increase in incidentally detected findings. These findings, generated primarily by cross-sectional imaging studies, have significant downstream cost implications. Furthermore, concerns over the economic burden of incidental findings can influence policy decisions to either approve or decline reimbursement for new imaging technologies and applications, as in the case of CTC for colorectal cancer screening.[21,42]

Published cost data relevant to imaging-detected incidental findings are sparse and do not yet enable accurate estimation of the economic burden of imaging-detected incidental findings in the current health care system.[18] Substantial further work is needed in this field. Although further primary data collection is critical for better defining the scope of incidental findings and understanding current practice patterns related to their work up, the resource requirements for identifying the long-term costs, risks, and benefits of incidental findings are preclusively high in most settings. As detailed in this review, economic modeling techniques can be used to more efficiently estimate the long-term downstream costs and patient outcomes that result from incidental findings and to understand the effects of incidental findings on the value of widely used diagnostic imaging strategies. This combined approach of primary data collection and economic modeling has the potential to yield high-quality evidence regarding the burden of imaging-detected incidental findings in a wide spectrum of clinical and patient scenarios. Equipped with such information, clinicians and policy makers alike will be able to make better decisions about the appropriateness of imaging procedures in future health care practices.

REFERENCES

1. Chin M, Mendelson R, Edwards J, et al. Computed tomographic colonography: prevalence, nature, and clinical significance of extracolonic findings in a community screening program. Am J Gastroenterol 2005;100(12):2771–6.

2. Flicker MS, Tsoukas AT, Hazra A, et al. Economic impact of extracolonic findings at computed tomographic colonography. J Comput Assist Tomogr 2008;32(4):497–503.

3. Gluecker TM, Johnson CD, Wilson LA, et al. Extracolonic findings at CT colonography: evaluation of prevalence and cost in a screening population. Gastroenterology 2003;124(4):911–6.

4. Veerappan GR, Ally MR, Choi JH, et al. Extracolonic findings on CT colonography increases yield of colorectal cancer screening. AJR Am J Roentgenol 2010;195(3):677–86.

5. Hara AK, Johnson CD, MacCarty RL, et al. Incidental extracolonic findings at CT colonography. Radiology 2000;215(2):353–7.

6. Kimberly JR, Phillips KC, Santago P, et al. Extracolonic findings at virtual colonoscopy: an important consideration in asymptomatic colorectal cancer screening. J Gen Intern Med 2009;24(1):69–73.

7. Pickhardt PJ, Hanson ME, Vanness DJ, et al. Unsuspected extracolonic findings at screening CT colonography: clinical and economic impact. Radiology 2008;249(1):151–9.

8. Tolan DJ, Armstrong EM, Chapman AH. Replacing barium enema with CT colonography in patients older than 70 years: the importance of detecting extracolonic abnormalities. AJR Am J Roentgenol 2007;189(5):1104–11.

9. Xiong T, McEvoy K, Morton DG, et al. Resources and costs associated with incidental extracolonic findings from CT colonography: a study in a symptomatic population. Br J Radiol 2006;79(948):948–61.

10. Yee J, Kumar NN, Godara S, et al. Extracolonic abnormalities discovered incidentally at CT colonography in a male population. Radiology 2005;236(2):519–26.

11. Liu W, Mortele KJ, Silverman SG. Incidental extraurinary findings at MDCT urography in patients with hematuria: prevalence and impact on imaging costs. AJR Am J Roentgenol 2005;185(4):1051–6.

12. Maizlin ZV, Barnard SA, Gourlay WA, et al. Economic and ethical impact of extrarenal findings on potential living kidney donor assessment with computed tomography angiography. Transpl Int 2007;20(4):338–42.

13. Yousem DM, Huang T, Loevner LA, et al. Clinical and economic impact of incidental thyroid lesions found with CT and MR. AJNR Am J Neuroradiol 1997;18(8):1423–8.

14. Kucharczyk MJ, Menezes RJ, McGregor A, et al. Assessing the impact of incidental findings in a lung cancer screening study by using low-dose computed tomography. Can Assoc Radiol J 2010. [Epub ahead of print].

15. Machaalany J, Yam Y, Ruddy TD, et al. Potential clinical and economic consequences of noncardiac incidental findings on cardiac computed tomography. J Am Coll Cardiol 2009;54(16):1533–41.

16. Lee CI, Tsai EB, Sigal BM, et al. Incidental extracardiac findings at coronary CT: clinical and economic impact. AJR Am J Roentgenol 2010;194(6):1531–8.

17. Baker LC, Atlas SW, Afendulis CC. Expanded use of imaging technology and the challenge of measuring value. Health Aff (Millwood) 2008;27(6):1467–78.

18. Smith-Bindman R, Miglioretti DL, Larson EB. Rising use of diagnostic medical imaging in a large integrated health system. Health Aff (Millwood) 2008;27(6):1491–502.

19. Orme NM, Fletcher JG, Siddiki HA, et al. Incidental findings in imaging research: evaluating incidence, benefit, and burden. Arch Intern Med 2010;170(17):1525–32.

20. Pearson SD, Knudsen AB, Scherer RW, et al. Assessing the comparative effectiveness of a diagnostic technology: CT colonography. Health Aff (Millwood) 2008;27(6):1503–14.

21. Zauber AG, Knudsen AB, Rutter CM, et al. Cost-effectiveness of CT colonography to screen for colorectal cancer: technology assessment report. Published 2009. Available at: http://www.cms.gov/determinationprocess/downloads/id58TA.pdf. Accessed December 6, 2010.

22. U.S. Preventive Services Task Force. Screening for colorectal cancer: U.S. Preventive Services Task Force recommendation statement. Ann Intern Med 2008;149(9):627–37.

23. Decision memo for screening computed tomography (CTC) for colorectal cancer (CAG-00396N). 2009. Available at: http://www.cms.gov/mcd/viewdecisionmemo.asp?from2=viewdecisionmemo.asp&id=220&. Accessed October 20, 2010.

24. Zalis ME, Barish MA, Choi JR, et al. CT colonography reporting and data system: a consensus proposal. Radiology 2005;236(1):3–9.

25. Central Intelligence Agency. The World Factbook. 2010. Available at: https://www.cia.gov/library/publications/the-world-factbook/fields/2076.html. Accessed October 20, 2010.

26. Messersmith WA, Brown DF, Barry MJ. The prevalence and implications of incidental findings on ED abdominal CT scans. Am J Emerg Med 2001; 19(6):479–81.

27. MacRedmond R, Logan PM, Lee M, et al. Screening for lung cancer using low dose CT scanning. Thorax 2004;59(3):237–41.

28. Black C, Bagust A, Boland A, et al. The clinical effectiveness and cost-effectiveness of computed tomography screening for lung cancer: systematic reviews. Health Technol Assess 2006;10(3):iii–iiv, ix–x, 1–90.

29. McMahon PM, Kong CY, Johnson BE, et al. Estimating long-term effectiveness of lung cancer screening in the Mayo CT screening study. Radiology 2008;248(1):278–87.

30. Mortensen JD, Woolner LB, Bennett WA. Gross and microscopic findings in clinically normal thyroid glands. J Clin Endocrinol Metab 1955;15(10):1270–80.

31. Sosnouski D, Bonsall RP, Mayer FB, et al. Extracardiac findings at cardiac CT: a practical approach. J Thorac Imaging 2007;22(1):77–85.

32. Knudsen AB, Lansdorp-Vogelaar I, Rutter CM, et al. Cost-effectiveness of computed tomographic colonography screening for colorectal cancer in the medicare population. J Natl Cancer Inst 2010; 102(16):1238–52.

33. Lee JM, McMahon PM, Kong CY, et al. Cost-effectiveness of breast MR imaging and screen-film mammography for screening BRCA1 gene mutation carriers. Radiology 2010;254(3):793–800.

34. Pandharipande PV, Gervais DA, Hartman RI, et al. Renal mass biopsy to guide treatment decisions for small incidental renal tumors: a cost-effectiveness analysis. Radiology 2010;256(3):836–46.

35. Weinstein MC, Siegel JE, Gold MR, et al. Recommendations of the panel on cost-effectiveness in health and medicine. JAMA 1996;276(15):1253–8.

36. Berland LL, Silverman SG, Gore RM, et al. Managing incidental findings on abdominal CT: white paper of the ACR incidental findings committee. J Am Coll Radiol 2010;7(10):754–73.

37. Lee JM, Kopans DB, McMahon PM, et al. Breast cancer screening in BRCA1 mutation carriers: effectiveness of MR imaging—Markov Monte Carlo decision analysis. Radiology 2008;246(3):763–71.

38. Hrung JM, Langlotz CP, Orel SG, et al. Cost-effectiveness of MR imaging and core-needle biopsy in the preoperative work-up of suspicious breast lesions. Radiology 1999;213(1):39–49.

39. Swan JS, Fryback DG, Lawrence WF, et al. MR and conventional angiography: work in progress toward assessing utility in radiology. Acad Radiol 1997; 4(7):475–82.

40. Swan JS, Sainfort F, Lawrence WF, et al. Process utility for imaging in cerebrovascular disease. Acad Radiol 2003;10(3):266–74.

41. Swan JS, Ying J, Stahl J, et al. Initial development of the temporary utilities index: a multiattribute system for classifying the functional health impact of diagnostic testing. Qual Life Res 2010;19(3): 401–12.

42. U.S. Preventive Services Task Force. Screening for colorectal cancer: recommendation and rationale. Ann Intern Med 2002;137(2):129–31.

Imaging of Incidental Findings on Thoracic Computed Tomography

Jeffrey B. Alpert, MD*, David P. Naidich, MD

KEYWORDS
- Incidental • Nodule • Thymoma

IMAGING OF INCIDENTAL FINDINGS ON THORACIC COMPUTED TOMOGRAPHY

Computed tomography (CT) of the chest remains one of the most commonly used tools in the assessment of thoracic disease. With continued technologic advancement of multidetector CT (MDCT), ultrathin 1 mm or less volumetric sections of the thorax can be obtained during a single breath-hold. As a result, with higher spatial resolution and greater overall sensitivity, MDCT of the chest has produced a greater number of findings, many of which are unsuspected and of uncertain clinical significance. Among nearly 200 CT angiograms performed in an emergency setting for assessment of pulmonary embolism, Hall and colleagues[1] found that patients were more than twice as likely to demonstrate a new incidental finding (24%) that required follow-up than pulmonary embolism (9%).

An incidental finding may be considered as any finding that is unsuspected or unrelated to the clinical indication for imaging. When discovered, incidental findings must be categorized as clinically significant or clinically insignificant. If significant, one must determine if immediate action should be taken (such as a newly discovered malignancy), if the finding needs to be recognized and reassessed in time (such as a nonspecific lung nodule), or if the finding needs to be recognized without further work-up (such as variant vascular anatomy).

Jacobs and colleagues[2] examined 11 screening studies for lung cancer and coronary artery disease and found a wide range of reported incidental thoracic findings. Lung cancer screening studies reported an average of 14.2% of patients with significant incidental findings, compared with 7.7% of patients undergoing coronary artery screening, a difference attributed to the limited field of view used on cardiac CT. There was considerable variation among all screening studies with unexpected findings that required follow-up, ranging from 3% to 41.5%. Furthermore, recommendations for further evaluation varied widely. These authors found that although there was consistency regarding the definitions used to classify incidental findings, there was a lack of uniformity regarding both the clinical significance and recommendations ascribed to the findings.

Although there are well-established guidelines for follow-up of some incidental findings such as small solid lung nodules, there is no clear follow-up algorithm for many other unexpected findings.[3] As a result, with an increasing number of incidental findings, there are now twice as many additional imaging studies recommended when compared to over 10 years ago.[4] This increase is often associated with additional exposure to ionizing radiation and likely a greater risk of radiation-induced malignancy. Ultimately, incidental findings can also become a significant source of medical cost, patient anxiety, and confusion. This article discusses and illustrates

No grant funding or other support was provided for this work.
Thoracic Imaging Section, Department of Radiology, NYU Langone Medical Center, 560 First Avenue, IRM 236, New York, NY 10016, USA
* Corresponding author.
E-mail address: Jeffrey.Alpert@downstate.edu

Radiol Clin N Am 49 (2011) 267–289
doi:10.1016/j.rcl.2010.10.005
0033-8389/11/$ – see front matter © 2011 Elsevier Inc. All rights reserved.

the spectrum of the most commonly encountered incidental findings on thoracic CT studies, as well as attempts to differentiate those for which additional imaging or clinical correlation is required from those for which additional evaluation is unwarranted.

LUNG

The discovery of a small unsuspected lung nodule on chest CT is among the most frequent indications for follow-up imaging of an incidental finding. In aforementioned study by Hall and colleagues,[1] an incidental pulmonary nodule was identified in 22% of 589 CT pulmonary angiograms; in 13% of patients, the nodule was a new finding that required follow-up imaging. In a review of several coronary artery screening studies, Jacobs and colleagues[2] noted that pulmonary nodules were one of the most common significant incidental findings seen in a wide range (0.44%–19%) of subjects, illustrating an ongoing debate in current literature regarding whether or not such findings should be followed or even reported.[5,6]

When discovered unexpectedly on CT and no prior imaging studies exist to document 2-year stability, solid lung nodules may demonstrate characteristic features that are reassuring for benignity, therefore sparing the patient unnecessary radiation exposure in the form of multiple follow-up studies. A nodule that demonstrates fat attenuation, for instance, is consistent with a lung hamartoma, the most common benign neoplasm of the lung that is seen most commonly in middle-aged adult men (Fig. 1).[7] Hamartomas are unencapsulated, lobulated lesions that are reported to contain fat attenuation in up to 50% of cases.[7,8] When fat is present, an attenuation measurement of −40 to −120 HU is a reliable indicator of hamartoma, provided there is no history of fat-containing malignancy such as liposarcoma or renal cell carcinoma.[9] Hamartomas are also composed of fibrous tissue, epithelial components, and cartilage that produces chondroid calcification in 5% to 50% of subjects.[7,8,10] This "popcorn" pattern of calcification is thought to convey a benign cause. Diffuse, central, or lamillated nodule calcifications are also traditionally thought to reflect benignity in patients without underlying malignancy, whereas some patients with osteosarcoma, for example, may demonstrate calcified metastatic nodules.[11] Indeterminate patterns such as eccentric, stippled, or amorphous calcifications are not reliably categorized as benign or malignant.

In association with lung cancer screening studies, several investigators have attempted to illustrate other nodule characteristics that are predictive of benign behavior. It must be emphasized, however, that these studies were performed among screening populations without underlying malignancy, and therefore, these trends are not to be directly applied to the general population. Among nearly 900 noncalcified 5- to 10-mm nodules identified on lung cancer screening CT and followed over 1 year, Xu and colleagues[12] identified no malignancy among nodules that were smooth with attachments to vessels, pleura, or fissures. Among other nodules, nodule size was the best predictor of malignancy. Ahn and colleagues[13] discovered that 28% of nodules detected on lung cancer screening chest CT were perifissural: these were often triangular (44%), oval (42%), and inferior to the carina (84%), with a septal connection (73%) and a mean maximal length of 3.2 mm (Fig. 2). None of these nodules developed into cancer over 7 years of follow-up,

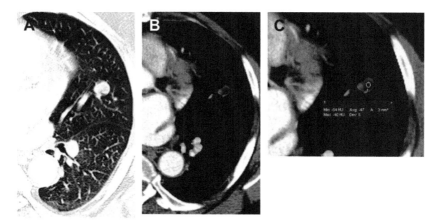

Fig. 1. Axial images viewed in high- and low-frequency window settings (A, B) demonstrating left upper lobe nodule. (C) Region-of-interest mean attenuation of nearly −50 HU is consistent with fat, confirming the presence of hamartoma.

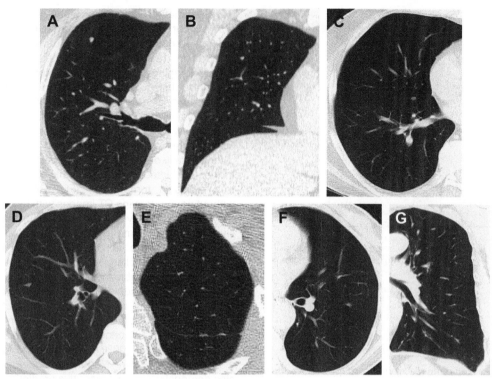

Fig. 2. (*A*, *B*) A perifissural nodule is seen corresponding to the horizontal fissure on axial and coronal images. (*C*) A rectangular nodule is seen in the region of the right oblique fissure. (*D*, *E*) Triangular nodules correspond to the oblique fissures in 2 patients. (*F*, *G*) Axial and coronal images of a triangular nodule associated with the left oblique fissure.

even among the small number of perifissural nodules (7 of 159) that initially increased in size and then remained stable. These findings suggest that the malignant potential of these perifissural nodules is low. In addition to peripheral subpleural location, Takashima and colleagues[14] found that nodules detected on lung cancer screening CT, which were predominantly solid attenuation and polygonal in shape, were commonly benign. Nodules with a 3-dimensional ratio greater than 1.78 had 100% specificity for benignity among 72 characterized nodules measuring 1 cm or less. Over time, Takashima and colleagues[15] discovered that lesion regression or polygonal shape were the most sensitive predictors of benignity, whereas nodule growth and ground-glass opacity were the most sensitive for malignancy.

Several studies have suggested that subpleural nodules may represent intrapulmonary lymph nodes (**Fig. 3**).[16,17] Shaham and colleagues,[17] for instance, retrospectively described CT characteristics of nodules in 18 patients with cytology-proven intrapulmonary lymph nodes. These nodules were typically solid, homogeneous, well defined, and often oval, round, triangular, or trapezoidal in shape. These lymph nodes were all seen below the level of

the carina with a median size of 5.8 mm, and one-third of these demonstrated a thin pleural tag. Although subpleural nodules are increasingly recognized as intrapulmonary lymph nodes, CT imaging is unable to determine the pathologic characteristics of the node in question.

Among nonscreening populations, lung nodules demonstrate a higher incidence of malignancy. Benjamin and colleagues[18] found that 11% of unsuspected nodules less than 1 cm were malignant when followed over time, although among patients without known cancer, the malignancy rate may be as low as 1%. Among 254 patients with a single lung nodule who underwent video-assisted thoracoscopic surgery and resection, 55% of nodules were malignant, although 77% (108 of 140) of malignant nodules were present in patients with known malignancy.[19]

Ultimately, recommendations of the Fleischner Society guide appropriate follow-up of small unsuspected lung nodules, based primarily on nodule size and patient risk factors. The group recommends more aggressive workup of nodules greater than 8 mm in size, as these nodules are associated with a higher likelihood of malignancy; 18% of nodules measuring 8 to 20 mm in size and

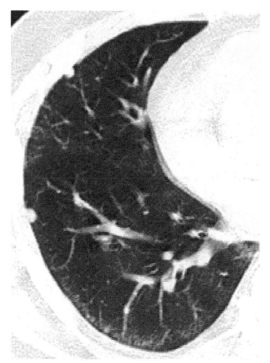

Fig. 3. Well-defined, round, subpleural nodules discovered unexpectedly on chest CT. Tissue sampling confirmed the presence of intrapulmonary lymph nodes.

50% of nodules measuring greater than 20 mm are thought to be malignant.[3,20–22] Although these recommendations do not apply to patients with underlying malignancy, the group also notes that factors such as patient age and comorbid disease should be part of the decision-making process when considering overall lung cancer risk.

Although a recent study has found that Fleischner Society guidelines are well known among radiologists, there are varying degrees of conformity to these guidelines, with a higher rate of conformity seen among those in academic practice, with at least one radiologist with specialized thoracic fellowship training, and among those practicing fewer than 5 years.[23] Ultimately, clinical management of these incidental nodules relies on several other factors, including not only malignancy risk factors but also the risks and benefits of further investigation and, of course, patient preference.[24] With an ever increasing number of CT examinations performed in the United States, both the medical community and the public has become increasingly aware of the cumulative ionizing radiation dose accrued from numerous diagnostic and screening studies.[25–27] However, it has been shown that many radiologists and clinicians tend to underestimate the additive effects of ionizing radiation.[28]

Several radiation dose–saving techniques are available without compromising image quality, including automated dose modulation and breast shielding. In addition, radiologists should be prepared to modify imaging protocols to promote low-dose technique using decreased kVp for both CT pulmonary angiography and lung cancer screening, as well as imaging only the portion of the thorax involved when performing repeated follow-up studies, when appropriate.

Incidentally detected solid lung nodules may be further evaluated with fluorodeoxyglucose–positron emission tomography (FDG-PET) with or without accompanying CT images with high accuracy, thus potentially reducing the number of invasive procedures among patients with nonavid, presumably benign solid nodules (Fig. 4).[29,30] Christensen and colleagues[31] reported that PET imaging was preferable to another characterization technique called nodule-enhancement CT, based on the greater specificity of PET (76% vs 29%). However, these authors maintain that nodule-enhancement CT technique is a valuable tool, with a sensitivity of 100% (PET was found to have a sensitivity of 96%). Nodule-enhancement CT also demonstrates a high negative predictive value

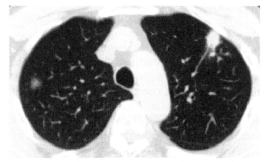

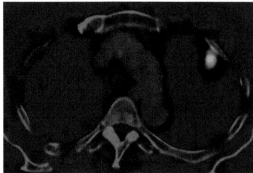

Fig. 4. Spiculated, irregular left upper lobe nodule (top) that demonstrates FDG-avidity on corresponding PET imaging (bottom). Note the ground-glass right upper lobe nodule, which fails to accumulate radiopharmaceutical, a pathologically proved focus of bronchoalveolar cell carcinoma.

(100%), greater patient convenience, and lower overall cost. With this technique, a nodule is considered malignant when there is an attenuation difference greater than 15 HU between unenhanced and peak contrast-enhanced images (Fig. 5). As previously suggested, if interest is limited to a solitary nodule, one should consider limiting the area included on the pre- and postcontrast data set, or any follow-up chest CT, to reduce unneeded radiation exposure.

Increased understanding of the significance of incidental lung nodules is not limited to solid nodules. The implications and management strategies of ground-glass and subsolid nodules are the discussions of many recent items in the literature. To accurately characterize subsolid nodules, one must use contiguous thin-section CT images (on the order of 1–3 mm) to thoroughly examine the nodular opacity for the presence of solid components that may be missed on routine 5-mm sections.

Kim and colleagues[32] determined that 6% of persistent ground-glass nodules represented atypical adenomatous hyperplasia when examined histopathologically, 75% represented bronchoalveolar cell carcinoma (BAC) or adenocarcinoma with BAC, and 19% represented organizing pneumonia or nonspecific lung fibrosis. Unfortunately, no imaging features were identified to reliably differentiate among these causes (Fig. 6).

As described by Godoy and Naidich,[33] the size of pure ground-glass nodules provides important information that influences follow-up strategy. In keeping with the pathologic and CT imaging correlations of Noguchi, an isolated pure ground-glass nodule smaller than 5 mm in size is likely a small focus of atypical adenomatous hyperplasia (AAH). Although the presence of BAC is difficult to completely exclude, the very long doubling time of such malignancy suggests that follow-up imaging is probably unnecessary, especially among elderly patients. Nodules between 5 and 10 mm with pure ground-glass opacity should be reassessed in 3 to 6 months to determine if the opacity has resolved after antibiotic therapy, for instance, as such a lesion may represent a focus of infection, inflammation, or hemorrhage. If persistent, the ground-glass nodule may represent AAH or BAC, and although invasive adenocarcinoma may rarely be present within such a lesion, long-term follow-up imaging is preferred over surgical biopsy. Follow-up of a ground-glass nodule should persist longer than the 2 years often suggested to document benignity among solid nodules, as the lepidic growth pattern of bronchoalveolar carcinoma is associated with a long doubling time; significant differences in mean volume doubling time were found among pure ground-glass nodules (813 days), ground-glass and solid nodules (457 days), and solid nodules (149 days).[34]

In some instances, multiple ground-glass nodules are identified, which are more frequently seen among women and nonsmokers and more frequently composed of AAH and BAC rather than invasive adenocarcinoma.[35] Management of solitary and multiple nodules is similar, as prognoses are not significantly different. As such, management guidelines proposed by Godoy suggest a minimum of 3 consecutive annual follow-up studies to document stability. Furthermore, as previously suggested, if a solitary nodule is being reassessed on follow-up imaging, low-dose CT limited to the region of interest should be considered to reduce cumulative radiation dose delivered by numerous follow-up CT examinations.

Regarding part-solid nodules, Noguchi and colleagues'[36] classification scheme indicates that solid components within otherwise ground-glass nodules represent structural collapse of normal architecture, with fibroblast proliferation and stromal invasion corresponding to an element of

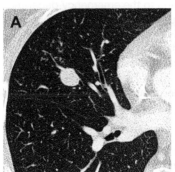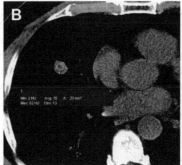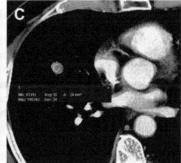

Fig. 5. (A) Thin-section 1-mm axial section illustrating middle lobe nodule with associated airway obstruction. Contrast-enhancement CT was performed; pre- and postcontrast images (B, C) in mediastinal windows illustrate enhancement of the nodule, measuring mean HU of 35 and 81 before and after contrast administration, respectively. This nodule was pathologically proved to represent carcinoid.

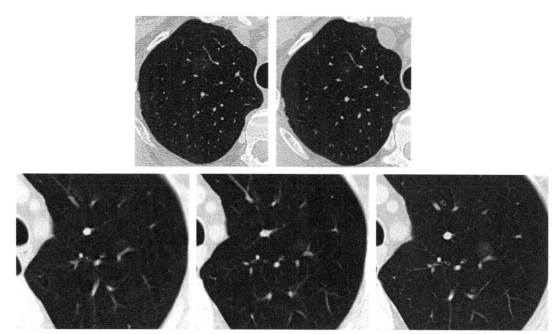

Fig. 6. (*Top*) Ground-glass right upper lobe nodule (*left*), unchanged 3 months later (*right*). Although nonspecific, a focus of bronchoalveolar cell carcinoma is suspected. (*Bottom*) Small ground-glass nodule originally thought to represent atypical adenomatous hyperplasia (*left*). Follow-up images 3 and 6 years later (*center, right*) illustrate increased size and conspicuity of the nodule, consistent with small bronchoalveolar cell carcinoma.

invasive adenocarcinoma (Fig. 7). When discovered incidentally, a part-solid nodule is nonspecific in etiology, and if the nodule is related to infection, hemorrhage, or other consolidative material, it may decrease in size or resolve on follow-up imaging. A recent article by Lee and colleagues[37] retrospectively studied the clinical and CT features of transient part-solid nodules identified on screening thin-section chest CT to determine predictive factors that may differentiate them from persistent part-solid nodules. The study found that 69.8% of 126 part-solid nodules were transient, and there were significant differences between transient and persistent part-solid nodules. Lesion multiplicity, large solid component, and ill-defined nodular border on thin-section CT were independent predictors of transient part-solid nodules, as were young patient age and serum eosinophilia. This study found that part-solid nodules with characteristics of transient behavior may be safely reassessed with short-term follow-up imaging without further intervention, even among nodules greater than 1 cm in size, despite the higher malignancy rate of part-solid nodules reported previously.[38]

Although PET is limited in the assessment of pure BAC, often producing false-negative results, it demonstrates greater sensitivity among mixed type adenocarcinoma (see Fig. 7). PET or PET/CT is also useful in such cases because metastatic spread is more likely with an invasive adenocarcinoma component. Regarding subsolid nodules, evaluation with PET imaging is preferred over surgical biopsy, as small foci of invasive adenocarcinoma may easily be missed by a relatively small biopsy specimen.[33]

Both the Early Lung Cancer Action Project and Anti-Lung Cancer Association screening programs have reported a low incidence of unexpected lung cancers among screening subjects, 0.7% and 0.37%, respectively.[39,40] Although the mean size of malignant lesions ranged from 12.4 to 15 mm between these 2 studies, the large majority of these cases were stage I disease. Even among nonscreening populations, the incidence of unsuspected lung cancer is low, occurring in 0.45% of patients presenting to the emergency department undergoing evaluation for pulmonary embolism, as reported by Kino and colleagues[41] (Fig. 8). However, in distinction to screening populations, these newly discovered lung cancers were typically advanced at presentation, categorized as stage IIIB or IV at the time of diagnosis.

AIRWAYS

In a review of incidental findings reported among several screening studies, airway abnormalities were infrequently reported to be less than 1%.[2] Although incidental findings corresponding to airways may be focal or diffuse, accurate assessment requires thin-section high-resolution CT

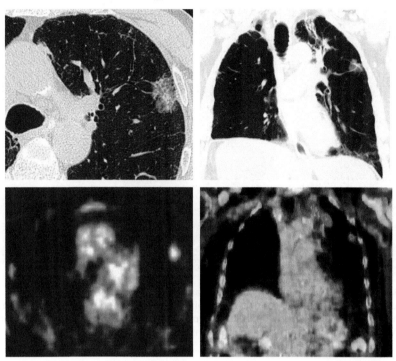

Fig. 7. (*Top*) Axial and coronal CT images reveal a subsolid left upper lobe nodule with both ground-glass and solid components. The nodule demonstrates FDG avidity on corresponding axial and coronal PET images (*bottom*). At surgery, adenocarcinoma with bronchoalveolar cell carcinoma features was identified.

technique. Contiguous 1-mm or smaller sections can be used to better visualize not only solid and subsolid lung nodules but also focal endobronchial abnormalities (Fig. 9). Select high-resolution ultra-thin sections, typically 1 mm each 10 mm, are also helpful in assessing regional or diffuse airway disease such as bronchiectasis or bronchial wall thickening. In those subjects in whom air trapping is suspected, expiratory high-resolution images should be used to accentuate the heterogeneous, geographic mosaic pattern of attenuation produced by obstructive airway disease (Fig. 10).

Air trapping is not uncommonly seen among patients with bronchial wall thickening, regardless of the underlying cause of airway disease. Regarding bronchial wall thickening, Nakano and colleagues[42] examined 22 patients with mild chronic obstructive pulmonary disease undergoing lung resection and found that CT-based dimensions of larger airways directly correlated with distal airway obstruction demonstrated histologically. There has been varied discussion on this topic, including differences among patients with asthma, smoking history, and other causes of airway inflammation. However, recently, Copley and colleagues[43] described bronchial wall thickening in up to 60% of individuals older than 75 years (vs 6% of individuals younger than 55 years),

regardless of pack-year smoking history, suggesting that this finding may also be related to senescent changes of the lung. After reviewing thin-section chest CT of asymptomatic elderly patients and their younger counterparts, Copley and colleagues[43] also described a greater incidence of limited, predominantly subpleural basal reticulation and

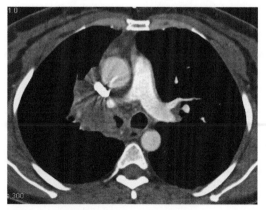

Fig. 8. Contrast-enhanced axial image in a patient presenting to the emergency department with suspected pulmonary embolism. A large right hilar mass was unexpectedly discovered.

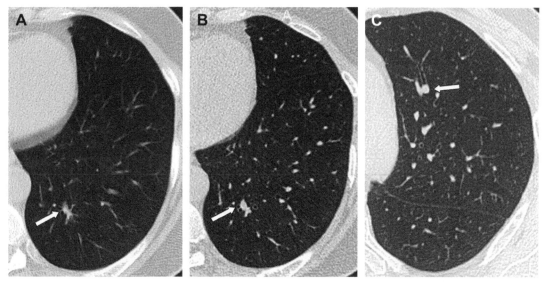

Fig. 9. (A) On 7-mm axial images, a branching pulmonary vessel is seen in the left lower lobe. (B) Thin-section 1-mm images better illustrate the presence of a 3-mm solid perivascular lung nodule, which is not well visualized on thick-section images. (C) Thin-section 1-mm image in a different patient showing a nodular opacity within a segmental airway. In this patient, the nodule represented focal mucoid impaction.

thin-walled lung cysts (identified among 60% and 25% of older individuals, respectively, vs none of the younger cohort).

Retained secretions are one of the most frequently seen abnormalities of large caliber airways. Secretions may seem globular, strand like, or may layer dependently within the airway lumen (Fig. 11). While demonstrating soft tissue attenuation on CT, a discrete filling defect within the airway is often nonspecific. Foci of air within the area are helpful in establishing a benign cause, although direct bronchoscopic inspection or follow-up imaging may be needed to exclude neoplasia. Other focal abnormalities such as tracheal bronchus are usually more straightforward (Fig. 12).

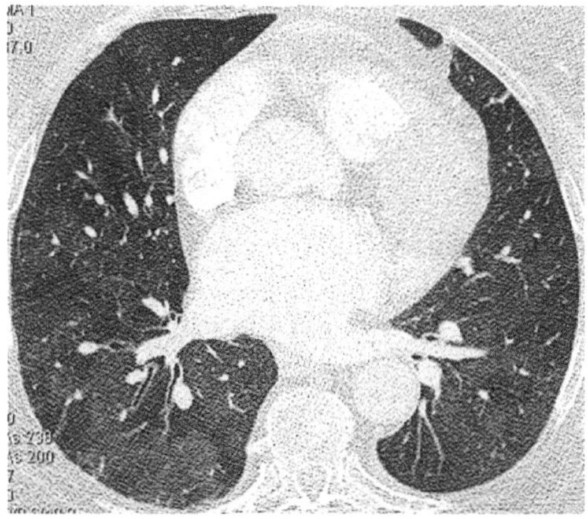

PLEURA

Incidental abnormalities of the pleura are most commonly pleural effusions, followed by focal abnormalities such as noncalcified or calcified pleural plaques.[2,44] Clinically significant incidental pleural abnormalities, namely indeterminate pleural masses, were rarely reported among lung cancer screening studies in less than 1% of subjects.[2]

When incidentally discovered on CT, imaging characteristics may provide definitive evaluation of pleural lesions. Pleural lipoma, for instance, may arise from the pleura or the extrapleural space but should demonstrate homogeneous fat attenuation on CT, measuring −50 to −150 HU with few linear strands of fibrous stroma (Fig. 13).[7,45]

Soft tissue–attenuation pleural lesions may reflect benign or malignant disease. Localized fibrous tumors of the pleura are uncommon lesions often discovered incidentally among adults in the sixth and seventh decades of life.[46–49] When symptomatic, the lesion is associated with hypertrophic pulmonary osteoarthropathy and hypoglycemia in 35% and 4% of subjects, respectively.[47] Up to 37% of fibrous tumors are histologically malignant, although all benign and up to half of all malignant lesions are successfully managed with surgical

Fig. 10. Thin-section axial image, illustrating a mosaic lung attenuation pattern consistent with mild air trapping. Mild bronchial wall thickening is also identified in the right lower lobe.

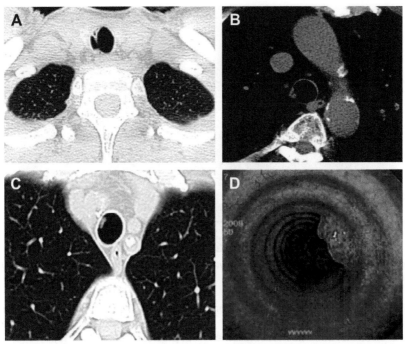

Fig. 11. (*A*) Strand-like opacity within the tracheal lumen, illustrating retained secretions. Foci of air are reassuring for a benign cause. (*B*) Nodular soft tissue material adjacent to the lateral wall of the trachea may reflect retained secretions, although other causes cannot be excluded. Mediastinal lipomatosis is incidentally noted. (*C, D*) Possible secretions seen on CT actually represent a tracheal papilloma, better characterized on bronchoscopy (Bronchoscopic image *courtesy of* Eric Leibert, MD, NYU Langone Medical Center).

excision. Arising from the visceral pleura in 80% of cases, fibrous tumors are typically well defined, spherical or ovoid lesions, which measure soft tissue attenuation on CT (Fig. 14). These lesions are often pedunculated, which is virtually pathognomonic for diagnosis, and may be mobile when examined under fluoroscopy. On magnetic resonance imaging (MRI), these enhancing lesions are typically low-signal intensity on T1-weighted images and high-signal intensity on T2-weighted images, related to a high degree of cellularity.[47]

Whether solitary or multiple, the large majority of pleural neoplasms represent metastatic disease, commonly from lung (40%), breast (20%), gastrointestinal or pelvic malignancies (30%), or lymphoma (10%).[47,49] Uncommonly, invasive thymoma may produce multiple pleural masses, although if discovered incidentally, one may expect to see an

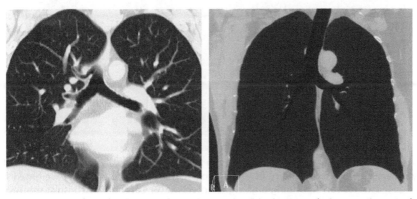

Fig. 12. Reformatted coronal and minimum-intensity projection images demonstrating tracheal bronchus supplying the right upper lobe.

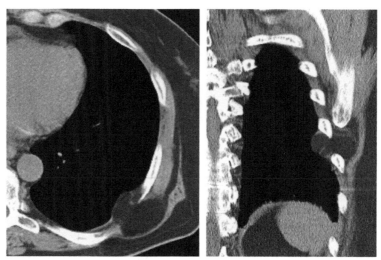

Fig. 13. Axial and coronal images in low-frequency window setting reveal a lipoma with both pleural and extrapleural components.

anterior mediastinal mass or evidence of prior surgery, suggesting recurrent thymoma.

Diffuse pleural diseases, such as mesothelioma and lymphoma, must also be considered when mass-like pleural abnormalities are identified, and frequently, tissue sampling is required for definitive diagnosis. Contrast administration is valuable for accurate assessment of the presence and extent of pleural disease (Fig. 15).

Occasionally, it is uncertain if an unsuspected mass arises from the pleura or the adjacent tissues of the posterior mediastinum (Fig. 16). Visualization

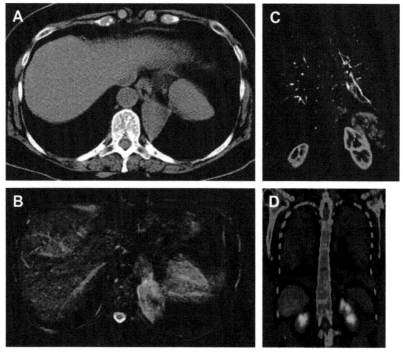

Fig. 14. (*A*) Axial noncontrast CT image demonstrating a triangular soft tissue mass at the medial left lung base, pathologically proven to represent solitary fibrous tumor of the pleura. (*B*) Axial T2-weighted magnetic resonance (MR) image illustrates corresponding high-signal intensity. (*C*) Coronal postcontrast subtraction MR image demonstrates enhancement of the solitary fibrous tumor, whereas corresponding coronal PET/CT image (*D*) reveals no significant FDG avidity.

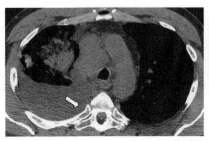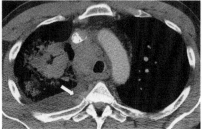

Fig. 15. Although not a true incidental image, in this patient with known lung cancer these pre- and postcontrast axial images viewed in mediastinal windows illustrate improved visualization of nodular posterior right pleural thickening after intravenous contrast administration.

of a pleural fat plane is required to accurately document a pleural origin of the mass. However, in some instances, such as those with neurogenic tumors arising from the paraspinal or posterior mediastinal regions, it may be difficult to differentiate between pleural and paraspinal fat. Although neurogenic tumors are described later in this article, it should be noted that MRI characteristics are often nonspecific, and tissue sampling may be needed for definitive evaluation.

MEDIASTINUM

Incidental mediastinal masses are rare, with a reported prevalence of less than 1% of asymptomatic individuals at high risk for lung cancer undergoing

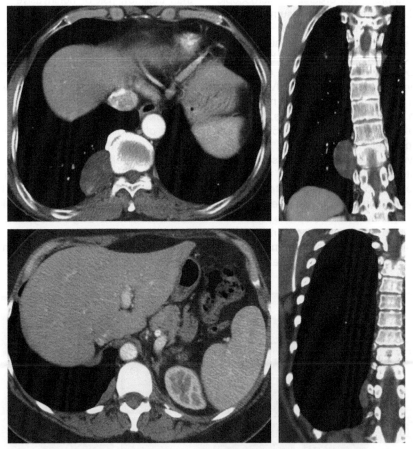

Fig. 16. (*Top*) Axial and coronal postcontrast images demonstrating a right paraspinal mass, pathologically proved to represent schwannoma, abutting the lateral margin of the vertebral body and neural foramen. (*Bottom*) Axial and coronal postcontrast images illustrating foci of right pleural thickening, attributed to pleural involvement of invasive thymoma.

screening CT.[50] Henschke and colleagues[50] reported that most incidental mediastinal masses were of thymic origin (with an overall prevalence of 0.45%), 20% of which were smaller than 3 cm in size and were unchanged 1 year later.

The thymus typically reaches its maximum relative size during the first few months of life and its maximum absolute size during puberty, only to involute and undergo fatty replacement (Fig. 17).[51,52] Early work by Baron and colleagues[53] characterized the normal-appearing thymus on 154 CT studies and found that the thymus was visible in 73% of patients aged 30 to 49 years and 17% of patients older than 49 years. The thymus is sensitive to stressors such as infection, surgery, neoplasia, and chemotherapy and may shrink to 40% of its original size. However, as the body recovers, the thymus regains its original size and may grow up to 50% greater in size, referred to as thymic rebound hyperplasia.[51,52] Thymic rebound hyperplasia can be seen in 10% to 25% of patients undergoing chemotherapy, for instance.[54] True thymic hyperplasia suggests preserved organized microscopic features, and the thymus usually assumes an oval shape with diffuse enlargement and a smooth contour with a mixture of fat and soft tissue attenuation on CT. In contrast, lymphoid thymic hyperplasia is often associated with autoimmune disease or early human immunodeficiency virus (HIV) infection, and although the thymus maintains its normal size and shape in nearly 50% of individuals, the gland may become enlarged or nodular in 35% or 20% of cases, respectively.[51]

On MRI, thymic tissue is homogeneous with signal intensity greater than that of muscle on T1-weighted images and similar to fat on T2-weighted images. Thymic tissue is usually not well seen on PET imaging but may show avid FDG uptake in rebound hyperplasia, which may be alarming for more worrisome causes like thymic carcinoma or lymphoma. In such instances, correlation with clinical history is vitally important.

Thymoma is a benign or low-grade malignant tumor arising from thymic epithelium, composed of immature nonneoplastic T cells. Thymomas, the most common primary anterior mediastinal neoplasm in adults, comprise 20% of all mediastinal neoplasms with a peak incidence within the fifth and sixth decades of life.[51,52,55] These lesions are usually asymptomatic, although paraneoplastic syndromes such as myasthenia gravis are seen in 30% to 50% of subjects with thymoma, and hypogammaglobulinemia and red cell aplasia are present in 10% and 5% of patients, respectively. On CT, thymomas are typically homogeneous, well circumscribed, round, or oval soft tissue masses that do not conform to the arrowhead or bilobed shape or concave margins of the normal thymus (Fig. 18). Up to one-third of lesions may demonstrate necrosis, hemorrhage, or cystic change, typically when enlarged.[55] Calcification of the mass or capsule may be present in approximately 22% of subjects and is thought to be more common among high-risk or invasive thymomas than their low-risk or noninvasive counterparts.[56] Although thymomas are completely encapsulated, approximately 30% demonstrate invasion of the tumor capsule with extension into surrounding mediastinal fat, and although invasive thymoma lacks the histologic features of malignancy seen among thymic carcinomas, these aggressive lesions may involve the pleura, lung, pericardium, or cardiovascular structures.

It is often difficult to determine if thymoma is invasive or noninvasive based on CT imaging. Jeong and colleagues[56] hoped to describe CT findings that correlated with histopathologic subtypes of thymoma and found that although there is limited correlation between imaging characteristics and histologic subtypes outlined by the World Health Organization (WHO), lobulated or irregular contour was more commonly seen in high-risk thymomas and thymic carcinomas compared with low-risk thymomas. The authors

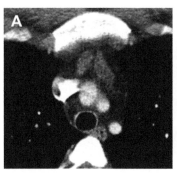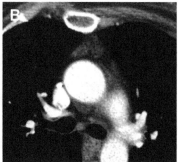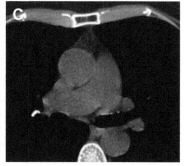

Fig. 17. Normal-appearing thymus in 3 patients. (*Left*) Bilobed, V-shaped appearance of the thymus in a 19-year-old man. (*Center, right*) Although thymic tissue is still visible in these 47- and 68-year-old patients, there is evidence of increasing fatty replacement.

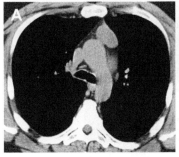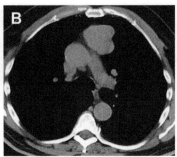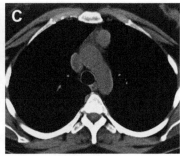

Fig. 18. Round, lobulated soft tissue in the anterior mediastinum in 3 patients, consistent with thymoma. Although CT is often limited in its ability to determine aggressive behavior, invasion of adjacent mediastinal fat (*right*) is a highly worrisome finding.

also determined that these qualities, as well as invasion of mediastinal fat or great vessels or pleural involvement, conveyed a higher chance of recurrent disease. On MRI, thymoma typically demonstrates intermediate signal intensity on T1-weighted images and increased signal on T2-weighted images.[51,52] In comparison to CT, MRI can be a useful tool in the assessment of adjacent tissue and vessel invasion, especially when contrast agent is administered. Chemical shift artifact may also be used to differentiate thymic masses such as thymoma from thymic hyperplasia, as hyperplasia will demonstrate decreased signal intensity on opposed-phase imaging.[57]

Although management of thymoma remains controversial, complete surgical excision is usually attempted, especially among lesions approaching 3 cm, because of the propensity for tumor recurrence and increased difficulty of resection of larger tumors.[50,58] Although prognosis is directly related to Masaoka tumor stage and WHO histologic classification, complete surgical excision has been shown to correlate with improved long-term survival.[59,60] Radiation and chemotherapy may also be administered based on stage of disease. Long-term follow-up imaging is advised to monitor for tumor recurrence.[58]

Thymic cysts are less common thymic lesions that may be congenital or acquired.[51,52] Congenital cysts arise from embryologic remnants of the thymopharyngeal duct, extending from the upper neck to the anterior mediastinum. Acquired cysts are often associated with chemotherapy, prior thoracotomy, or patients with associated thymoma. Although thymic cysts are commonly unilocular, multilocular cysts are associated with HIV infection and are now reported less frequently because of increased use of retroviral medication. Regardless of cause, thymic cysts are well-circumscribed, homogeneous lesions with thin, occasionally calcified walls (Fig. 19). No solid components or contrast

enhancement should be present; if present, thymoma with cystic change should be considered. Thymolipoma is another rare, benign thymic lesion comprising 5% of thymic neoplasms.[51,52] These lesions are encapsulated and pliable, conforming to adjacent mediastinal structures. With no age or sex predilection, these lesions are typically asymptomatic and are therefore often discovered incidentally. Imaging is usually sufficient for confident diagnosis of thymolipoma; the lesion demonstrates predominantly fat attenuation on CT, with strands of fibrous septa and thymic tissue (Fig. 20). High-signal intensity is seen on both T1- and T2-weighted MRI sequences, with strands of lower signal intensity corresponding to soft tissue septa.

Although uncommon, extragonadal germ cell tumors are most frequently found in the anterior mediastinum.[7,55,61] Eighty percent of these lesions are benign teratomas, which are commonly asymptomatic. Although there is no sex predilection,

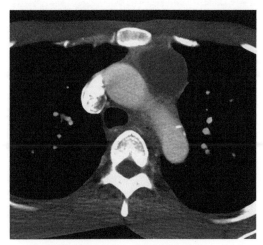

Fig. 19. An incidentally discovered thymic cyst. No nodular enhancing soft tissue component is appreciated on this postcontrast axial image.

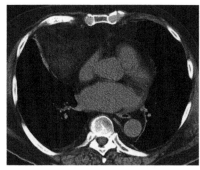
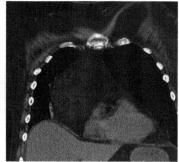

Fig. 20. Axial and coronal images of an unsuspected thymolipoma, producing mild mass effect on right atrium. Strands of soft tissue extend from the anterior mediastinum to the right cardiophrenic border.

benign teratomas are most commonly seen among young adults and may produce symptoms related to mass effect when large. Lesions are typically well circumscribed, round or oval, and lobulated, demonstrating a combination of cystic components, fat attenuation, and calcification in 88%, 76%, and 53% of masses, respectively.[55,61] Composed of all 3 germinal cell layers, teratomas may contain teeth, bone, or calcification in up to 20% of subjects.[7] The presence of a fat-fluid level, although rare, is highly specific. The appearance of teratoma on MRI corresponds to the heterogeneous composition of the lesion, and capsular rim enhancement may be appreciated on contrast-enhanced studies.

The thyroid gland is seen inconsistently on thoracic CT, and there is a wide reported range of incidental thyroid abnormalities between 0.5% and 16.8%.[44,62] Although a heterogeneous thyroid goiter may be the most commonly expected thyroid abnormality identified on CT (Fig. 21), Yoon and

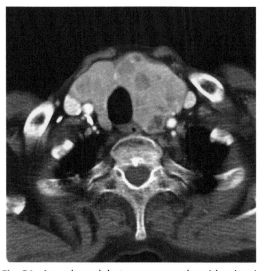

Fig. 21. An enlarged, heterogeneous thyroid goiter is one of the most recognizable incidental thyroid abnormalities.

colleagues[62] found that 12.5% of incidental thyroid nodules detected on CT were malignant. They described CT characteristics that suggested malignancy such as nodular or rim calcification, anterior-posterior to transverse measurement ratio greater than 1.0 and mean attenuation value greater than 130 on contrast-enhanced CT. The thyroid is commonly further assessed with sonography, which also allows opportunity for fine-needle aspiration, if appropriate.

In a study of the prevalence of incidental findings on CT pulmonary angiography, Hall and colleagues[1] found that 9% of cases demonstrated new adenopathy that required further follow-up. These cases included adenopathy greater than 1 cm in short axis not associated with parenchymal consolidation, nodes larger than 3 cm, or multiple enlarged mediastinal or hilar nodes.[1] The presence of nodal calcification is important to recognize and may assist in determining the significance of the finding. Regardless, incidental adenopathy is frequently nonspecific, and correlation with both lung parenchymal findings and the patient's medical history are necessary. PET/CT may be considered to assess associated metabolic activity and if uncertainty persists, surgical or transbronchial tissue sampling may be needed for more definitive evaluation.

As previously mentioned, the presence of a posterior mediastinal or paraspinal lesion such as neurogenic tumor may be difficult to differentiate from a primary pleural mass (see Fig. 16). Posterior mediastinal neurogenic tumors arising from neural elements are classified by their tissue of origin and may be malignant or benign; lesions arising from intercostal nerves, such as neurofibroma or schwannoma, are the most frequently seen neurogenic tumors among adults. These lesions are round or oval paravertebral soft tissue masses that may produce tumor extension into the spinal canal through an enlarged intervertebral foramen, forming a characteristic dumbbell shape. On CT, these lesions demonstrate soft tissue attenuation and may produce areas of heterogeneous attenuation due to cystic change or calcification.[63] Given their nonspecific appearance, MRI can be used for further assessment of these lesions: masses are of typically equal or slightly greater intensity than muscle on T1-weighted images and high-signal intensity on T2-weighted images. These neurogenic tumors demonstrate avid contrast enhancement; although when large, cystic changes may result in a heterogeneous appearance. Neurofibromas may demonstrate a characteristic target sign of central low signal surrounded by high-signal intensity on T2-weighted images.[63] However, it is often difficult to diagnose such lesions based on CT and MRI alone, and tissue sampling may be needed for definitive diagnosis.

CARDIOVASCULAR FINDINGS

Aortic disease accounts for most of the unsuspected cardiovascular findings on thoracic CT; aortic aneurysm was reported in up to 3.4% of patients undergoing lung cancer screening.[2] Such a finding is of variable significance, depending on the degree of aneurysmal enlargement. Surgical intervention should be considered when the thoracic aorta measures about 5.5 cm or greater in diameter or between 4 and 5 cm when the patient has an underlying connective tissue disease, such as Marfan, Ehlers-Danlos, or Turner syndromes, placing the patient at higher risk of an acute aortic syndrome.[64–67] If the aorta measures greater than 4 cm in diameter, follow-up CT or MRI is suggested in 6 months to assess interval growth. If the aneurysm has increased by more than 0.5 cm per year, surgery is suggested even if the vessel measures less than 5.5 cm, due to an increased risk of rupture.[67]

Although CT of the chest for suspected pulmonary embolism results in a large number of incidental findings, in some patients, pulmonary embolism itself may be an unexpected diagnosis (Fig. 22). With an annual incidence between 300,000 and 600,000 per year, pulmonary embolism is a well-recognized cause of substantial morbidity and mortality.[41] However, the incidental detection of pulmonary embolism on contrast-enhanced CT is an uncommon occurrence. Earlier studies by Gosselin and colleagues[68] and Winston and colleagues[69] describe an incidence of pulmonary embolism of 1.5% among all patients imaged, the large majority occurring among inpatients and among patients with cancer. However, more recent studies report an incidence of nearly 4% of patients, the vast majority of whom continue to be inpatients with malignancy.[70] These unexpected

pulmonary emboli are initially reported by the interpreting radiologist in only 25% of patients because of the small size of the pulmonary arteries that are affected.[71] On a related note, this increased incidence is presumably related to the technologic advances of MDCT, allowing improved visualization of distal pulmonary arteries. There has also been discussion regarding the incidental detection of thrombus within pulmonary artery stumps after pneumonectomy; Kwek and Wittram[72] found that 12.4% of 89 pneumonectomy patients had evidence of pulmonary artery stump thrombosis and that there was a direct relationship between stump length and likelihood of thrombus (see Fig. 22). Although only one patient was treated with anticoagulation for concomitant pulmonary embolism to the contralateral vasculature, none of the stump thrombi propagated, suggesting a benign natural history.

In adults, developmental vascular anomalies are unlikely to produce clinical symptoms but may be important to recognize in preparation of surgery or other intervention. Layton and colleagues[73] report that there are more than 20 different configurations of the aortic arch, the most common being the traditional branching pattern of 3 vessels arising directly from the arch, seen in 70% of patients. The most common variant occurs when the left common carotid artery shares a common origin with the innominate artery, resulting in 2 great vessels arising from the aortic arch, seen in 13% of patients (Fig. 23). Although this is commonly referred to as a bovine arch, or a bovine-type arch when the left common carotid artery originates from the innominate artery 1 to 2.5 cm from the arch, Layton and colleagues[73] contend that a true bovine aortic arch bears no resemblance to any common human aortic arch variant and is thus a misnomer. Aberrant right subclavian artery is another common variant, with an incidence of 1% to 2%.[74] Less commonly, a right aortic arch configuration is seen among 0.1% of the general population and may be related to other anomalies, depending on the branching pattern of the great vessels.[75] Although a right aortic arch with aberrant left subclavian artery is associated with developmental cardiac anomalies in 5% to 10% of patients (see Fig. 23), a mirror image branching pattern is almost always associated with congenital heart disease, most commonly tetralogy of Fallot, in 98% of patients and is unlikely to be incidentally discovered in an asymptomatic adult.[76]

Central venous anomalies involving the superior vena cava (SVC) or pulmonary veins may be easily overlooked on unenhanced chest CT, but variants of the SVC, for instance, are important to recognize

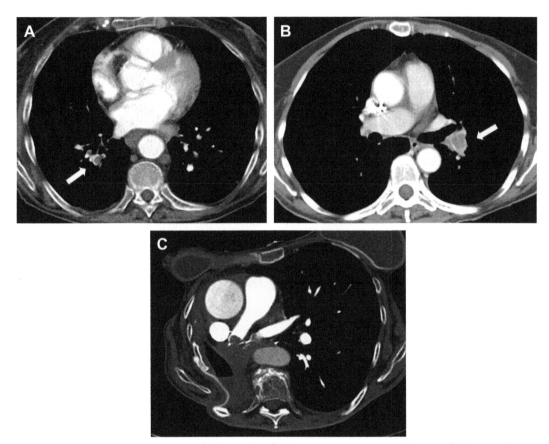

Fig. 22. (*A, B*) Incidental pulmonary embolism, identified in 2 asymptomatic patients with history of treated malignancy. (*C*) While undergoing CT to evaluate right bronchopleural fistula after pneumonectomy (see air-fluid level), thrombus was unexpectedly identified within the stump of the right pulmonary artery.

before intervention such as placement of permanent pacemaker or central venous catheter. Both dual and solitary left-sided SVC result from persistence of the left anterior cardinal vein, which commonly regresses during normal embryologic development.[77,78] Dual SVC is the most common congenital anomaly of the SVC, occurring in 0.3% to 0.5% of the general population and 4% of patients with congenital heart disease (Fig. 24).[77,78] Although dual SVC can be associated with atrial or ventricular septal defect, aortic coarctation, tetralogy of Fallot, or pulmonary stenosis, it is commonly an isolated anomaly in the adult. When both right-sided and left-sided SVCs are present, the right is smaller than the left in 65% of subjects.[78] The left-sided SVC drains into the coronary sinus in 90% of cases (Fig. 25), and in 10% of subjects, the left-sided SVC drains directly into the left atrium resulting in a right-to-left shunt, although this is associated with congenital heart disease and is rarely seen among adults with normally developed hearts.[77]

Partial anomalous pulmonary venous return (PAPVR) is an another uncommon anomaly representing abnormal drainage of one or more pulmonary veins into the systemic venous system such as the brachiocephalic vein, SVC or inferior vena cava, or right atrium (Fig. 26). The anomaly is reported in 0.04% of post-mortem studies, and although it has traditionally been considered more common on the right, Ho and colleagues[79] found that among 47 subjects, anomalous drainage of the left upper lobe was the most common variant in 47% of cases, followed by right upper lobe (38%), right lower lobe (13%), and left lower lobe (2%). Ho and colleagues found a prevalence of 0.1% in adults and speculated that the abnormality is likely underreported because of the absence of associated symptoms in adults, as well as the limited ability to differentiate between pulmonary and systemic vessels on noncontrast CT imaging. Although in children, PAPVR often presents with symptoms related to other congenital malformations such as sinus venosus atrial septal defect

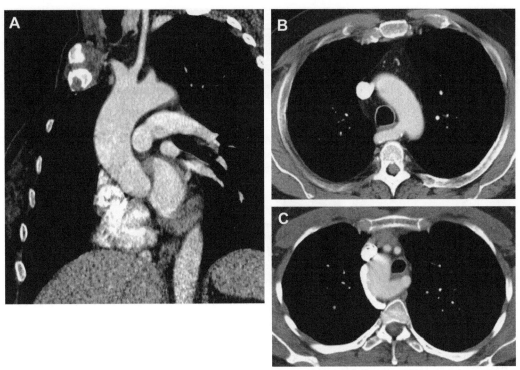

Fig. 23. Variant aortic anatomy. (*A*) The innominate and left common carotid arteries share a common origin in this patient with what is typically referred to as a bovine aortic arch. (*B*) Aberrant right subclavian artery arises from the aortic arch and passes posterior to the trachea. (*C*) Patient with right-sided aortic arch showing an anomalous origin of the left subclavian artery. In this adult patient, the incidentally discovered vascular anomaly was an isolated finding.

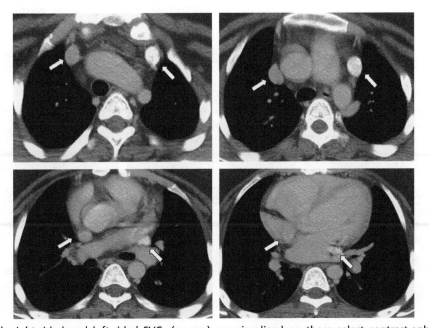

Fig. 24. Both right-sided and left-sided SVCs (*arrows*) are visualized on these select contrast-enhanced axial images. Intravenous contrast was delivered via the left upper extremity with resulting enhancement of the left-sided SVC.

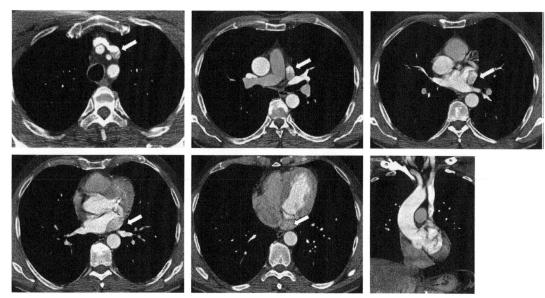

Fig. 25. Select contrast-enhanced axial and coronal (*bottom right*) images illustrate left-sided SVC, coursing toward the right atrium (*arrows*). A right-sided SVC is absent.

(which is most commonly associated with right upper lobe PAPVR), adults commonly have few or no associated abnormalities.

Other developmental venous anomalies involve the azygos vein, producing the characteristic azygos fissure, for instance (Fig. 27). Although uncommon, pulmonary vein varix may simulate a lung nodule or adenopathy on noncontrast images.[80]

CHEST WALL

Although discovered unexpectedly by the radiologist, many chest wall anomalies are easily recognized by the clinician before imaging. Chest wall deformities such as pectus excavatum and, less commonly, pectus carinatum are easily identified on routine axial images of the thorax (Fig. 28). Pectus excavatum, recognized when the ribs protrude anteriorly greater than the sternum, results in

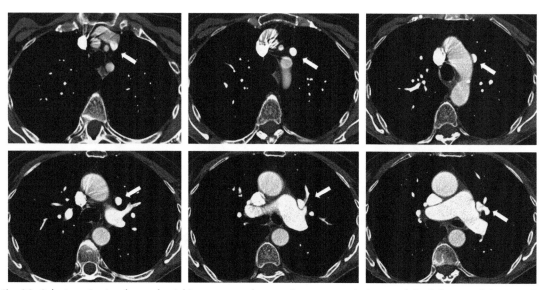

Fig. 26. Select contrast-enhanced axial images reveal anomalous venous drainage of the left upper lobe into the innominate vein (*arrows*). Recent literature has described partial anomalous pulmonary venous return of the left upper lobe as the most common form of this developmental anomaly.

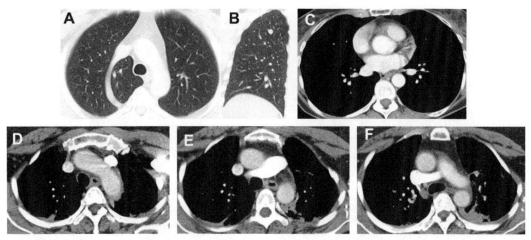

Fig. 27. (*A*, *B*) Axial and coronal images in high-frequency window setting illustrate the characteristic appearance of an azygos fissure. (*C*) Focal dilatation of the right inferior pulmonary vein. Venous varices such as this can sometimes be mistaken for lung nodule on chest radiography. (*D–F*) Three contrast-enhanced axial images showing anomalous course of the subaortic left innominate vein, passing inferior to the aortic arch.

a decreased anterior-posterior diameter of the thoracic cavity, often displacing the heart to the left. Surgical correction may be performed when severe, characterized by a transverse diameter to anterior-posterior diameter ratio of greater than 3.25, as described by Haller and colleagues.[81] In subjects with pectus carinatum, the sternum protrudes anteriorly, and although this may be

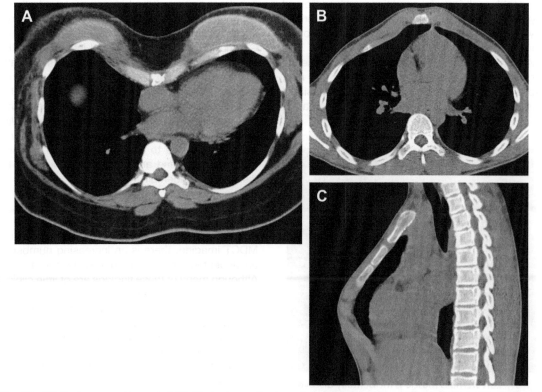

Fig. 28. (*A*) Pectus excavatum and (*B*, *C*) pectus carinatum deformities of the chest wall. Note the leftward displacement of the heart in the young woman with pectus excavatum.

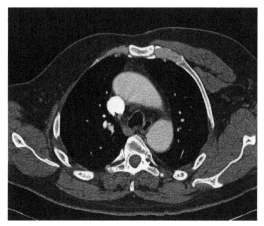

Fig. 29. The absence of right pectoralis major and minor muscles was incidentally noted in this patient with Poland syndrome, who obtained CT of the pulmonary arteries for suspicion of pulmonary embolism. Coincidentally, the patient was a Polish man who presented to the emergency department with shortness of breath and pleuritic chest pain after a flight from his home country.

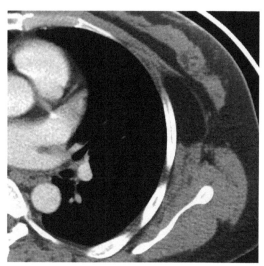

Fig. 31. Well-encapsulated, fat density lesion associated with the left serratus anterior muscle is consistent with chest wall lipoma, the most common benign chest wall neoplasm.

associated with congenital heart disease in younger patients, it may be an isolated anomaly in the adult.[82]

The radiologist is probably not the first physician to identify multifactorial conditions such as Poland syndrome, an uncommon condition characterized by partial or total absence of the greater pectoralis muscle and ipsilateral syndactyly (Fig. 29).[82] This syndrome may also be associated with absence or atrophy of ipsilateral second through fifth ribs, absence of the pectoralis minor, and aplasia of ipsilateral breast/nipple. Although less apparent

on physical examination, accessory muscles such as sternalis muscles may also be identified on CT (Fig. 30).

Regarding unexpected chest wall masses, lipoma is the most common benign soft tissue neoplasm and may have both intra- and extrathoracic components (Fig. 31).[82] These lesions demonstrate relatively homogeneous fat attenuation on CT and high T1-weighted signal intensity on MRI, and the presence of inhomogeneous nonfatty tissue should raise the possibility of malignancy such as liposarcoma.[82] The most common malignant neoplasms of the chest wall are fibrosarcoma and malignant fibrohistiocytoma. However, malignant neoplasms usually produce clinical symptoms such as pain due to their typically rapid, invasive growth pattern and are therefore less likely to be discovered incidentally.

SUMMARY

With continued improvement of high-resolution MDCT imaging, there is an increasing number of unsuspected findings identified in the thorax. Although many of these findings are of little clinical significance, others require additional imaging to exclude more worrisome causes, often resulting in greater exposure to ionizing radiation, increased cost, and patient anxiety. There is great variation among radiologists regarding what constitutes a clinically significant incidental thoracic finding, and there is often limited conformity regarding follow-up recommendations. As the definition of an incidental finding depends on the clinical

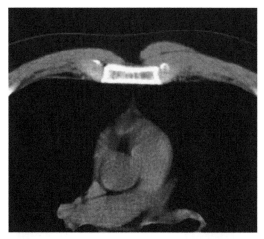

Fig. 30. Left sternalis muscle is incidentally discovered anterior to the left pectoralis major muscle in this young adult man.

indication for imaging, the findings described in this article are by no means exhaustive. However, the lack of clear follow-up guidelines for many conditions suggests that in some areas, further investigation is needed.

ACKNOWLEDGMENTS

The authors would like to express their gratitude to Drs Maj Wickstrom, Georgeann McGuinness, Gerri Brusca-Augello, Maria Shiau, Jane Ko, John Fantauzzi, Derek Mason, and David Pryluck for their valuable contributions.

REFERENCES

1. Hall WB, Truitt SG, Scheunemann LP, et al. The prevalence of clinically relevant incidental findings on chest computed tomographic angiograms ordered to diagnose pulmonary embolism. Arch Intern Med 2009;169(21):1961–5.
2. Jacobs PC, Mali WP, Grobbee DE, et al. Prevalence of incidental findings in computed tomographic screening of the chest: a systematic review. J Comput Assist Tomogr 2008;32(2):214–21.
3. MacMahon H, Austin JH, Gamsu G, et al. Guidelines for management of small pulmonary nodules detected on CT scans: a statement from the Fleischner Society. Radiology 2005;237(2):395–400.
4. Sistrom CL, Dreyer KJ, Dang PP, et al. Recommendations for additional imaging in radiology reports: multifactorial analysis of 5.9 million examinations. Radiology 2009;253(2):453–61.
5. Budoff MJ. Ethical issues related to lung nodules on cardiac CT. AJR Am J Roentgenol 2009;192(3): W146, [author reply: W147].
6. Lazoura O, Vassiou K, Kanavou T, et al. Incidental non-cardiac findings of a coronary angiography with a 128-slice multi-detector CT scanner: should we only concentrate on the heart? Korean J Radiol 2010;11(1):60–8.
7. Gaerte SC, Meyer CA, Winer-Muram HT, et al. Fat-containing lesions of the chest. Radiographics 2002;22(Spec No):S61–78.
8. Hansen CP, Holtveg H, Francis D, et al. Pulmonary hamartoma. J Thorac Cardiovasc Surg 1992; 104(3):674–8.
9. Muram TM, Aisen A. Fatty metastatic lesions in 2 patients with renal clear-cell carcinoma. J Comput Assist Tomogr 2003;27(6):869–70.
10. Siegelman SS, Khouri NF, Scott WW Jr, et al. Pulmonary hamartoma: CT findings. Radiology 1986; 160(2):313–7.
11. O'Keefe ME Jr, Good CA, McDonald JR. Calcification in solitary nodules of the lung. Am J Roentgenol Radium Ther Nucl Med 1957;77(6):1023–33.
12. Xu DM, van der Zaag-Loonen HJ, Oudkerk M, et al. Smooth or attached solid indeterminate nodules detected at baseline CT screening in the NELSON study: cancer risk during 1 year of follow-up. Radiology 2009;250(1):264–72.
13. Ahn MI, Gleeson TG, Chan IH, et al. Perifissural nodules seen at CT screening for lung cancer. Radiology 2010;254(3):949–56.
14. Takashima S, Sone S, Li F, et al. Small solitary pulmonary nodules (< or = 1 cm) detected at population-based CT screening for lung cancer: Reliable high-resolution CT features of benign lesions. AJR Am J Roentgenol 2003;180(4):955–64.
15. Takashima S, Sone S, Li F, et al. Indeterminate solitary pulmonary nodules revealed at population-based CT screening of the lung: using first follow-up diagnostic CT to differentiate benign and malignant lesions. AJR Am J Roentgenol 2003; 180(5):1255–63.
16. Miyake H, Yamada Y, Kawagoe T, et al. Intrapulmonary lymph nodes: CT and pathological features. Clin Radiol 1999;54(10):640–3.
17. Shaham D, Vazquez M, Bogot NR, et al. CT features of intrapulmonary lymph nodes confirmed by cytology. Clin Imaging 2010;34(3):185–90.
18. Benjamin MS, Drucker EA, McLoud TC, et al. Small pulmonary nodules: detection at chest CT and outcome. Radiology 2003;226(2):489–93.
19. Ginsberg MS, Griff SK, Go BD, et al. Pulmonary nodules resected at video-assisted thoracoscopic surgery: etiology in 426 patients. Radiology 1999; 213(1):277–82.
20. Henschke CI, Naidich DP, Yankelevitz DF, et al. Early lung cancer action project: initial findings on repeat screenings. Cancer 2001;92(1):153–9.
21. Pastorino U, Bellomi M, Landoni C, et al. Early lung-cancer detection with spiral CT and positron emission tomography in heavy smokers: 2-year results. Lancet 2003;362(9384):593–7.
22. Swensen SJ, Jett JR, Hartman TE, et al. Lung cancer screening with CT: Mayo Clinic experience. Radiology 2003;226(3):756–61.
23. Eisenberg RL, Bankier AA, Boiselle PM. Compliance with Fleischner Society guidelines for management of small lung nodules: a survey of 834 radiologists. Radiology 2010;255(1):218–24.
24. Gould MK, Fletcher J, Iannettoni MD, et al. Evaluation of patients with pulmonary nodules: when is it lung cancer?: ACCP evidence-based clinical practice guidelines (2nd edition). Chest 2007; 132(Suppl 3):108S–30S.
25. Brenner DJ, Hall EJ. Computed tomography–an increasing source of radiation exposure. N Engl J Med 2007;357(22):2277–84.
26. Fazel R, Krumholz HM, Wang Y, et al. Exposure to low-dose ionizing radiation from medical imaging procedures. N Engl J Med 2009;361(9):849–57.

27. Huppmann MV, Johnson WB, Javitt MC. Radiation risks from exposure to chest computed tomography. Semin Ultrasound CT MR 2010;31(1):14–28.

28. Lee CI, Haims AH, Monico EP, et al. Diagnostic CT scans: assessment of patient, physician, and radiologist awareness of radiation dose and possible risks. Radiology 2004;231(2):393–8.

29. Fischer BM, Mortensen J, Hojgaard L. Positron emission tomography in the diagnosis and staging of lung cancer: a systematic, quantitative review. Lancet Oncol 2001;2(11):659–66.

30. Fischer BM, Mortensen J. The future in diagnosis and staging of lung cancer: positron emission tomography. Respiration 2006;73(3):267–76.

31. Christensen JA, Nathan MA, Mullan BP, et al. Characterization of the solitary pulmonary nodule: 18F-FDG PET versus nodule-enhancement CT. AJR Am J Roentgenol 2006;187(5):1361–7.

32. Kim HY, Shim YM, Lee KS, et al. Persistent pulmonary nodular ground-glass opacity at thin-section CT: histopathologic comparisons. Radiology 2007; 245(1):267–75.

33. Godoy MC, Naidich DP. Subsolid pulmonary nodules and the spectrum of peripheral adenocarcinomas of the lung: recommended interim guidelines for assessment and management. Radiology 2009; 253(3):606–22.

34. Hasegawa M, Sone S, Takashima S, et al. Growth rate of small lung cancers detected on mass CT screening. Br J Radiol 2000;73(876):1252–9.

35. Kim TJ, Goo JM, Lee KW, et al. Clinical, pathological and thin-section CT features of persistent multiple ground-glass opacity nodules: comparison with solitary ground-glass opacity nodule. Lung Cancer 2009;64(2):171–8.

36. Noguchi M, Morikawa A, Kawasaki M, et al. Small adenocarcinoma of the lung. Histologic characteristics and prognosis. Cancer 1995;75(12):2844–52.

37. Lee SM, Park CM, Goo JM, et al. Transient part-solid nodules detected at screening thin-section CT for lung cancer: comparison with persistent part-solid nodules. Radiology 2010;255(1):242–51.

38. Henschke CI, Yankelevitz DF, Mirtcheva R, et al. CT screening for lung cancer: frequency and significance of part-solid and nonsolid nodules. AJR Am J Roentgenol 2002;178(5):1053–7.

39. Henschke CI, McCauley DI, Yankelevitz DF, et al. Early lung cancer action project: a summary of the findings on baseline screening. Oncologist 2001;6(2):147–52.

40. Kaneko M, Kusumoto M, Kobayashi T, et al. Computed tomography screening for lung carcinoma in Japan. Cancer 2000;89(Suppl 11):2485–8.

41. Kino A, Boiselle PM, Raptopoulos V, et al. Lung cancer detected in patients presenting to the emergency department studies for suspected pulmonary embolism on computed tomography pulmonary angiography. Eur J Radiol 2006;58(1):119–23.

42. Nakano Y, Wong JC, de Jong PA, et al. The prediction of small airway dimensions using computed tomography. Am J Respir Crit Care Med 2005; 171(2):142–6.

43. Copley SJ, Wells AU, Hawtin KE, et al. Lung morphology in the elderly: comparative CT study of subjects over 75 years old versus those under 55 years old. Radiology 2009;251(2):566–73.

44. van de Wiel JC, Wang Y, Xu DM, et al. Neglectable benefit of searching for incidental findings in the Dutch-Belgian lung cancer screening trial (NELSON) using low-dose multidetector CT. Eur Radiol 2007;17(6):1474–82.

45. Epler GR, McLoud TC, Munn CS, et al. Pleural lipoma. Diagnosis by computed tomography. Chest 1986;90(2):265–8.

46. Briselli M, Mark EJ, Dickersin GR. Solitary fibrous tumors of the pleura: eight new cases and review of 360 cases in the literature. Cancer 1981;47(11): 2678–89.

47. Dynes MC, White EM, Fry WA, et al. Imaging manifestations of pleural tumors. Radiographics 1992; 12(6):1191–201.

48. England DM, Hochholzer L, McCarthy MJ. Localized benign and malignant fibrous tumors of the pleura. A clinicopathologic review of 223 cases. Am J Surg Pathol 1989;13(8):640–58.

49. Kuhlman JE, Singha NK. Complex disease of the pleural space: radiographic and CT evaluation. Radiographics 1997;17(1):63–79.

50. Henschke CI, Lee IJ, Wu N, et al. CT screening for lung cancer: prevalence and incidence of mediastinal masses. Radiology 2006;239(2):586–90.

51. Nasseri F, Eftekhari F. Clinical and radiologic review of the normal and abnormal thymus: pearls and pitfalls. Radiographics 2010;30(2):413–28.

52. Nishino M, Ashiku SK, Kocher ON, et al. The thymus: a comprehensive review. Radiographics 2006;26(2): 335–48.

53. Baron RL, Lee JK, Sagel SS, et al. Computed tomography of the normal thymus. Radiology 1982; 142(1):121–5.

54. Choyke PL, Zeman RK, Gootenberg JE, et al. Thymic atrophy and regrowth in response to chemotherapy: CT evaluation. AJR Am J Roentgenol 1987; 149(2):269–72.

55. Strollo DC, Rosado de Christenson ML, Jett JR. Primary mediastinal tumors. Part 1: tumors of the anterior mediastinum. Chest 1997;112(2):511–22.

56. Jeong YJ, Lee KS, Kim J, et al. Does CT of thymic epithelial tumors enable us to differentiate histologic subtypes and predict prognosis? AJR Am J Roentgenol 2004;183(2):283–9.

57. Takahashi K, Inaoka T, Murakami N, et al. Characterization of the normal and hyperplastic thymus on chemical-shift MR imaging. AJR Am J Roentgenol 2003;180(5):1265–9.

58. Vita ML, Tessitore A, Cusumano G, et al. Recurrence of thymoma: re-operation and outcome. Ann Ital Chir 2007;78(5):375–6.

59. Davenport E, Malthaner RA. The role of surgery in the management of thymoma: a systematic review. Ann Thorac Surg 2008;86(2):673–84.

60. Margaritora S, Cesario A, Cusumano G, et al. Thirty-five-year follow-up analysis of clinical and pathologic outcomes of thymoma surgery. Ann Thorac Surg 2010;89(1):245–52 [discussion: 252].

61. Moeller KH, Rosado-de-Christenson ML, Templeton PA. Mediastinal mature teratoma: imaging features. AJR Am J Roentgenol 1997;169(4):985–90.

62. Yoon DY, Chang SK, Choi CS, et al. The prevalence and significance of incidental thyroid nodules identified on computed tomography. J Comput Assist Tomogr 2008;32(5):810–5.

63. Tateishi U, Gladish GW, Kusumoto M, et al. Chest wall tumors: radiologic findings and pathologic correlation: part 1. Benign tumors. Radiographics 2003; 23(6):1477–90.

64. Elefteriades JA. Natural history of thoracic aortic aneurysms: indications for surgery, and surgical versus nonsurgical risks. Ann Thorac Surg 2002; 74(5):S1877–80 [discussion: S1892–8].

65. Hiratzka LF, Bakris GL, Beckman JA, et al. 2010 ACCF/AHA/AATS/ACR/ASA/SCA/SCAI/SIR/STS/SVM Guidelines for the Diagnosis and Management of Patients with Thoracic Aortic Disease. J Am Coll Cardiol 2010;55(14):e27–129.

66. Kouchoukos NT, Dougenis D. Surgery of the thoracic aorta. N Engl J Med 1997;336(26):1876–88.

67. Svensson LG, Kouchoukos NT, Miller DC, et al. Expert consensus document on the treatment of descending thoracic aortic disease using endovascular stent-grafts. Ann Thorac Surg 2008;85(Suppl 1): S1–41.

68. Gosselin MV, Rubin GD, Leung AN, et al. Unsuspected pulmonary embolism: prospective detection on routine helical CT scans. Radiology 1998;208(1): 209–15.

69. Winston CB, Wechsler RJ, Salazar AM, et al. Incidental pulmonary emboli detected at helical CT: effect on patient care. Radiology 1996;201(1):23–7.

70. Storto ML, Di Credico A, Guido F, et al. Incidental detection of pulmonary emboli on routine MDCT of the chest. AJR Am J Roentgenol 2005;184(1):264–7.

71. Gladish GW, Choe DH, Marom EM, et al. Incidental pulmonary emboli in oncology patients: prevalence, CT evaluation, and natural history. Radiology 2006; 240(1):246–55.

72. Kwek BH, Wittram C. Postpneumonectomy pulmonary artery stump thrombosis: CT features and imaging follow-up. Radiology 2005;237(1):338–41.

73. Layton KF, Kallmes DF, Cloft HJ, et al. Bovine aortic arch variant in humans: clarification of a common misnomer. AJNR Am J Neuroradiol 2006;27(7): 1541–2.

74. Karcaaltincaba M, Haliloglu M, Ozkan E, et al. Non-invasive imaging of aberrant right subclavian artery pathologies and aberrant right vertebral artery. Br J Radiol 2009;82(973):73–8.

75. Yasuda T, Yamamoto S, Ishida Y. Double aneurysms of arch and descending aorta associated with right aortic arch. Ann Thorac Surg 2000;70(4):1405–7.

76. Kirks DR, Griscom NT, editors. Practical pediatric imaging: diagnostic radiology of infants and children. 3rd edition. Philadelphia: Lippincott-Raven; 1998. p. 581–3.

77. Burney K, Young H, Barnard SA, et al. CT appearances of congential and acquired abnormalities of the superior vena cava. Clin Radiol 2007;62(9): 837–42.

78. Demos TC, Posniak HV, Pierce KL, et al. Venous anomalies of the thorax. AJR Am J Roentgenol 2004;182(5):1139–50.

79. Ho ML, Bhalla S, Bierhals A, et al. MDCT of partial anomalous pulmonary venous return (PAPVR) in adults. J Thorac Imaging 2009;24(2):89–95.

80. Vanherreweghe E, Rigauts H, Bogaerts Y, et al. Pulmonary vein varix: diagnosis with multi-slice helical CT. Eur Radiol 2000;10(8):1315–7.

81. Haller JA Jr, Kramer SS, Lietman SA. Use of CT scans in selection of patients for pectus excavatum surgery: a preliminary report. J Pediatr Surg 1987; 22(10):904–6.

82. Jeung MY, Gangi A, Gasser B, et al. Imaging of chest wall disorders. Radiographics 1999;19(3):617–37.

Hepatic Incidentalomas

Richard M. Gore, MD*, Geraldine M. Newmark, MD,
Kiran H. Thakrar, MD, Uday K. Mehta, MD,
Jonathan W. Berlin, MD

KEYWORDS

- Incidentaloma • Hepatic cyst • Bile duct hamartoma
- Hepatic hemangioma • Focal nodular hyperplasia
- Hepatic adenoma • Liver metastases • Liver CT

Recent advances in multidetector computed tomography (MDCT), magnetic resonance (MR) imaging, and ultrasonography have led to the detection of incidental hepatic lesions in both the oncology and nononcology patient population that in the past remained undiscovered. These incidentalomas are unexpected, asymptomatic abnormalities that are discovered serendipitously while searching for other pathology.[1–18] Such incidental hepatic lesions have created a management dilemma for both clinicians and radiologists, particularly in the oncology patient in whom any mass, clinical or subclinical, warrants further evaluation. Strategies for optimizing patient management of these lesions are only beginning to emerge in terms of deciding which of these incidentalomas can be ignored, which can simply be monitored over time, and which require more aggressive workup.

Subjecting the patient to unnecessary testing and treatment carries its own set of risks that can result in an injurious and expensive cascade of imaging and intervention. Preoperative fine-needle aspiration may minimize diagnostic error but is associated with a nontrivial morbidity of 0.5% and mortality of 0.05%.[19] The exhaustive evaluation performed in some patients reflects the unwillingness of many physicians to accept uncertainty even in the case of a very rare diagnosis. This unwillingness is in part driven by a paucity of data on the topic, the lack of clear-cut algorithms with regard to diagnostic and treatment strategies, fear of potential malpractice liability, and/or the anxiety of the patient. In this review, guidelines concerning the approach to some of the more common hepatic incidentalomas are presented.

CYSTIC (ULTRASONOGRAPHY AND MDCT), HYPOINTENSE (T1-WEIGHTED MR IMAGING), AND HYPERINTENSE (T2-WEIGHTED) HEPATIC INCIDENTALOMAS

Hepatic lesions that are cystic on ultrasonography on MDCT, hypointense on T1-weighted MR imaging, and hyperintense on T2-weighted MR imaging are commonly found incidentally. Their differential diagnosis is extensive and they are usually benign in patients with no history of malignancy, hepatic dysfunction, or hepatic risk factors. These lesions are listed in Box 1 and are discussed more fully in this section.

Hepatic Cysts

Simple hepatic cysts are single, unilocular cysts that lined by a single layer of cuboidal bile duct epithelium. The walls of these cysts are composed of a thin layer of fibrous tissue adjacent to normal hepatic parenchyma. These cysts are considered to be congenital and developmental in origin, although they are typically discovered incidentally in the fifth through seventh decades of life.[20–22]

The incidence of simple hepatic cysts ranges up to 14% in autopsy series, 17% in CT series, and 20% in surgery series.[23,24] The vast majority of cysts are found incidentally and do not require

Department of Radiology, North Shore University Health System, Pritzker School of Medicine, University of Chicago, 2650 Ridge Avenue, Evanston, IL, USA
* Corresponding author. Department of Radiology, Evanston Hospital, 2650 Ridge Avenue, Evanston, IL 60201.
E-mail address: rgore@uchicago.edu

Radiol Clin N Am 49 (2011) 291–322
doi:10.1016/j.rcl.2010.10.004

any treatment or further evaluation. If sufficiently large, they can stretch Glisson's capsule leading to pain, cause biliary obstruction, or be complicated by hemorrhage or infection.[20–22]

Sonographically (Fig. 1A), simple hepatic cysts present as anechoic masses with smooth borders, nondetectable walls, no septations, no mural calcification, and posterior acoustic enhancement.[25]

On CT (see Fig. 1B), uncomplicated hepatic cysts manifest as well-defined, water-attenuated (<20 HU) intrahepatic masses, with smooth, thin walls, no internal structure, and no enhancement following contrast administration. The attenuation values of small hepatic cysts can be influenced by partial volume averaging, pixel size, matrix size, kilovoltage and milliamperage of the x-ray beam, slice thickness, reconstruction algorithm, patient diameter, and pseudoenhancement. All these factors can influence the attenuation of the cyst contents. Hemorrhage and infection can also lead to increased density of hepatic cysts.[20,23,24]

On MR (see Fig. 1C), cysts are usually oval-shaped, homogeneous, well-defined lesions that are sharply marginated with normal liver. Cysts have low signal intensity on T1-weighted images and high signal intensity on T2-weighted images; they do not show enhancement following contrast administration. Hemorrhage and infection can increase the signal intensity of cysts on T1-weighted images and can lead to inhomogeneity of the lesion.[26]

The differential diagnosis of a hepatic cyst includes cystic metastases from cystic primary tumors (ie, ovarian and cystic pancreatic primaries) and solid tumors that can produce cystic metastases (ie, gastrointestinal stromal tumor and endometrial carcinoma). Pyogenic and amebic abscesses typically show mural enhancement but can mimic cysts particularly when they are small. Cystic biliary neoplasms such as biliary cystadenoma or cystadenocarcinoma are usually large lesions with internal septations, mural nodularity, and a thicker wall.[27]

Bile Duct Hamartomas

Bile duct hamartomas (BDHs), also known as biliary microhamartomas or von Meyenburg complexes, are a focal disorderly collection of bile ducts that results from failure of involution of embryonic bile ducts. BDHs are composed of one or more dilated duct-like structures lined by biliary epithelium and accompanied by a variable amount of fibrous stroma. With extreme dilatation BDHs can be visible on cross-sectional imaging. BDHs range in size from 1 to 5 mm, and there can be 50,000 to 100,000 BDHs in a normal liver.[21] BDHs are found in 0.69% to 5.6% of individuals at autopsy.[21] BDHs as a rule are asymptomatic lesions found incidentally. Their major clinical significance is the fact that they may be misdiagnosed as multiple liver metastases or microabscesses.[28]

Virtually all persons with adult polycystic liver disease (APLD) have multiple BDHs and 11% of patients with multiple BDHs have APLD.[20,21] It is postulated that the larger cysts of APLD result from gradual dilatation of the hamartomas.

On cross-sectional imaging, BDHs are typically multiple round or irregular focal lesions of nearly uniform size (up to 15 mm) scattered throughout the liver.

Sonographically, BDHs have been described as either hypoechoic or anechoic small nodules with distal acoustic enhancement. However, hyperechoic biliary hamartomas or a combination of hypo- and hyperechoic lesions has also been reported. Small hyperechoic cystic lesions with comet-tail echoes may also be seen.[25–29]

BDHs manifest on CT (Fig. 2A, B) as multiple, widely scattered, small (<1.5 cm), low-attenuation lesions, which do not demonstrate discernible contrast enhancement.[24,30,31]

BDHs are hypointense on T1-weighted MR images (Fig. 3A) and hyperintense at T2-weighted images. If the TE (echo time) is increased at T2-weighted imaging, the signal intensity of these lesions increases further and approaches that of cerebrospinal fluid (see Fig. 3B, C). BDHs do not usually show contrast enhancement on CT or MR imaging, although

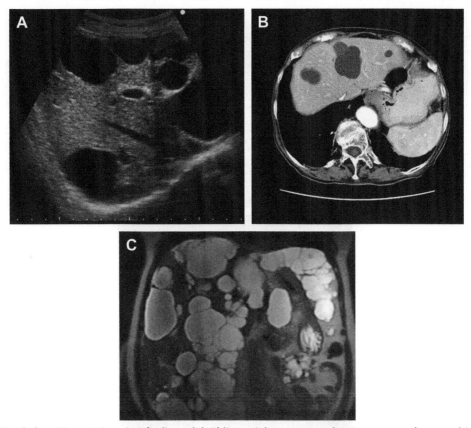

Fig. 1. Simple hepatic cysts: imaging findings. (*A*) Oblique right upper quadrant sonogram shows multiple well-marginated, thin-walled, anechoic hepatic cysts with increased through transmission of sound. (*B*) Axial contrast-enhanced CT scan shows large, bilateral, nonenhancing water density hepatic cysts. (*C*) Coronal T2-weighted MR image in a patient with adult polycystic liver and renal disease shows multiple well-marginated, hyperintense hepatic cysts with thin walls. Note the absence of mural thickening or nodularity.

a peripheral enhancing rim has been described on early and late postgadolinium images. Histopathologically, this rim enhancement correlates with compressed liver parenchyma surrounding the lesions.[32–34]

The differential diagnoses of BDHs include: metastatic disease, multiple microabscesses, Caroli disease, peribiliary cysts, primary sclerosing cholangitis, and simple hepatic cysts. BDHs are relatively uniform in size, whereas metastatic

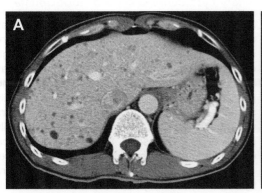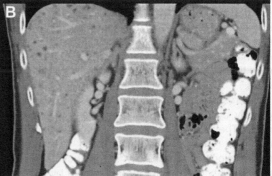

Fig. 2. Multiple bile duct hamartomas: CT features. Axial (*A*) and coronal (*B*) contrast-enhanced CT scans show innumerable tiny, nonenhancing cystic hepatic lesions.

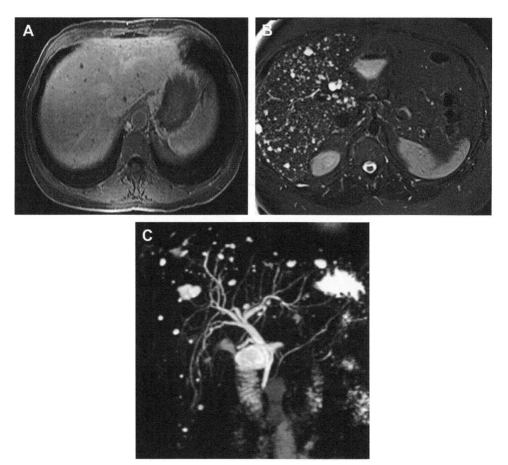

Fig. 3. Multiple bile duct hamartomas: MR features. (*A*) T1-weighted axial MR image demonstrates multiple, low signal-intensity cystic hepatic lesions. (*B*) T2-weighted image shows innumerable hyperintense cystic lesions. (*C*) MRCP image shows multiple tiny hyperintense cystic lesions.

lesions are usually more heterogeneous in size and in attenuation or signal intensity. Unlike BDHs, hepatic cysts are rarely as uniformly small or numerous, whereas the cysts in APLD are usually larger and more numerous.[35–37]

Polycystic Liver Disease

Patients with APLD are usually discovered incidentally at the time of radiologic examination. Approximately 70% of patients with APLD will also have polycystic kidney disease. Pathologically, these cysts are identical to simple cysts or BDHs.[21]

On cross-sectional imaging, APLD lesions are typically cystic and show no contrast enhancement. The lesions are well marginated and anechoic, and show increased through-transmission sonographically.[25] These cysts have water density on CT unless complicated by infection or hemorrhage. Mural calcification can occasionally be seen.[20,27] At MR imaging, cysts show

very low signal intensity on T1-weighted images and high signal intensity on T2-weighted images (see Fig. 1C). Higher signal intensity may be present on T1-weighted images as a result of hemorrhage or infection.[26,30]

Biliary Cystadenoma and Adenocarcinoma

Biliary cystadenomas and cystadenocarcinomas are rare cystic neoplasms lined by mucin-secreting columnar epithelium that are histologically and radiographically similar to cystadenomas and cystadenocarcinomas of the ovary and pancreas.[22] Biliary cystadenomas are usually seen in middle-aged women who may present with abdominal pain, distention, and occasionally jaundice.[20,25] When small, they may be seen incidentally and mimic benign hepatic cystic disease.

Sonographically, cystic biliary neoplasms are hypoechoic, and may have septations and a variable degree of mural thickening or nodularity.[20,25] On MDCT these lesions have low attenuation, and a unilocular or multilocular cystic appearance on CT (**Fig. 4**).[27]

Irregular papillary growths and mural nodules along the internal septa and wall are seen in cystadenomas and cystadenocarcinomas, although papillary excrescences and solid portions are more common in the latter. Cystadenomas occasionally have fine septal calcifications whereas cystadenocarcinomas may have thick, coarse, mural, and septal calcifications. The differential diagnosis of these lesions includes hepatic cysts, hydatid cysts, liver abscesses, cystic metastases, hematoma, cystic sarcomas, and choledochal cysts.[20,22,27]

Focal Hepatic Steatosis

Hepatic fatty metamorphosis or steatosis is the metabolic complication of a variety of toxic, ischemic, and infectious insults to the liver. It is the most common abnormality seen on liver biopsy of alcoholic patients and is observed in up to 50% of patients with diabetes. With the current obesity epidemic in the United States, hepatic steatosis is becoming increasingly common.[38]

When fatty infiltration is diffuse or lobar, segmental, or wedge shaped, differentiation from other focal hepatic disease is straightforward. In these cases the region of fat has a straight-line margin with normal parenchyma, typically extending to the liver capsule without associated bulging of the hepatic contour to suggest an underlying mass.[39,40]

When steatosis is nodular or focal, differentiation from metastatic disease and other masses can be problematic on CT.[41] Absolute CT attenuation values are unreliable indicators because fatty infiltration does not produce a fat-density lesion; rather, the steatosis merely diminishes the density of the region to lower than that of normal liver parenchyma.[42] There are several features that are helpful in this differentiation: focal fat does not cause local contour abnormalities; portal and hepatic venous branches course normally through the fatty areas; and these lesions may improve in a matter of days.[39]

The 2 most common areas of focal fatty infiltration and focal sparing in an otherwise normal or diffusely fatty liver are surrounding the gallbladder fossa and adjacent to the falciform ligament in segments II, III, and IV (**Figs. 5–7**). In the gallbladder fossa (**Fig. 8**), direct vascular communications to the portal system through aberrant gastric venous flow or accessory cystic veins permit perfusion of this portion of the liver by systemic blood flow rather than by splanchnic venous blood from the portal veins. The liver adjacent to the falciform ligament has also been shown to have aberrant direct venous flow. Consequently, a third blood supply to these areas may help spare them the adverse effects of toxic agents entering through the portal circulation. This variant vascular blood supply is also key in the development of regions of transient hepatic attenuation differences (THADs) on CT and transient hepatic intensity differences (THIDs) on MR imaging (see later discussion).[43]

On hepatic arterial phase (HAP) imaging, a hypovascular region is often seen in segment IV (**Fig. 9**) adjacent to the falciform ligament, which on portal venous phase (PVP) or delayed images becomes isodense with the liver. This appearance may result from the aberrant venous blood flow or from the fact that this region is a watershed area of hepatic arterial and portal venous blood flow.[39,43]

Sonographically, fat is hyperechoic due to an increased number of echogenic foci resulting from the proliferation of fat-nonfat interfaces. Four patterns of focal fatty hepatic infiltration have been described: hyperechoic nodule, multiple confluent hyperechogenic lesions, hypoechoic skip nodules, and irregular hyperechoic and hypoechoic areas. Focal areas of hepatic parenchyma may occasionally be spared from the fatty metamorphosis and appear as an ovoid, spherical, or sheet-like hypoechoic mass in an otherwise echogenic liver. Its characteristic location, the lack of mass effect on surrounding vessels, and a straight-line interface between normal and fatty parenchyma are useful differentiating signs.[25,39]

Hepatic hemangiomas (HH), which are typically hyperechoic compared with normal hepatic

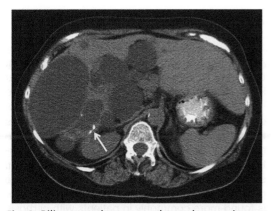

Fig. 4. Biliary cystadenomas and cystadenocarcinomas simulating multiple hepatic cysts: CT findings. Multiple hypodense lesions are identified within the liver are seen on this contrast-enhanced scan. One of the cystic lesions shows mural calcifications (*arrow*).

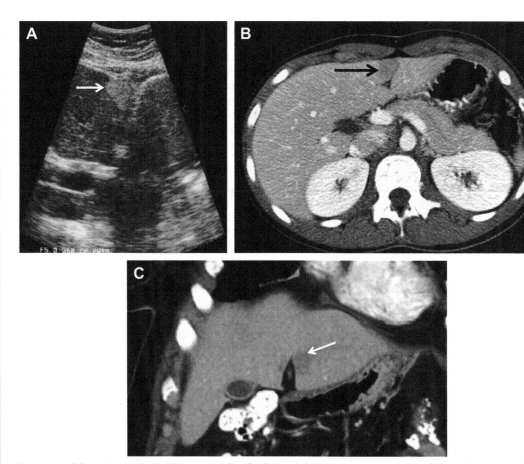

Fig. 5. Focal hepatic steatosis: CT-sonographic findings. (*A*) Transverse sonogram of the left lobe of the liver demonstrates a well-marginated, hyperechoic mass (*arrow*) in the medial segment of the left lobe adjacent to the falciform ligament. (*B*) Corresponding contrast-enhanced CT scan shows a hypodense "lesion" (*arrow*). (*C*) Coronal CT scan in a different patient shows focal fat (*arrow*) in the lateral segment of the left lobe.

parenchyma, may appear hypoechoic when compared with adjacent liver parenchyma in patients with a diffusely fatty liver, and MR or CT may be needed for differentiation.[44] Focal fatty infiltration in an otherwise normal-appearing liver on ultrasonography may also produce a hyperechoic space-occupying mass. An angular or interdigitating geometric margin is also characteristic of focal fat.[45]

MR imaging is particularly effective in evaluating the liver in patients with diffuse and focal steatosis. Proton chemical shift imaging, also termed opposed-phase gradient echo imaging, is a highly accurate technique in differentiating fatty metamorphosis from neoplasm. This technique exploits the difference in precession frequency between fat and water protons (3.37 ppm). On opposed-phase images, the fat signal is subtracted from the water signal whereas on in-phase images, the fat and water signals are combined. Lesions containing fat will therefore show a loss of signal intensity on the opposed-phase images when compared with the in-phase sequences.[46]

Fat Abutting the Intrahepatic Portion of the Inferior Vena Cava

A commonly seen, an incidental anatomic variant that simulates a mass is a focal collection of fat located medial to the intrahepatic portion of the inferior vena cava (IVC) at or above the level of confluence of the hepatic veins and the IVC. This fat is contiguous to the fat around the subdiaphragmatic portion of the esophagus. The fat collections have a characteristic location, orientation, size, shape, and density on CT (Fig. 10). The presence of this fat is not related to obesity but is found more commonly in patients with cirrhosis reflecting altered hepatic morphology. These fat collections should not be confused with hepatic fatty tumors such as lipoma, angiomyolipoma, or hepatic neoplasms, which often contain fat such

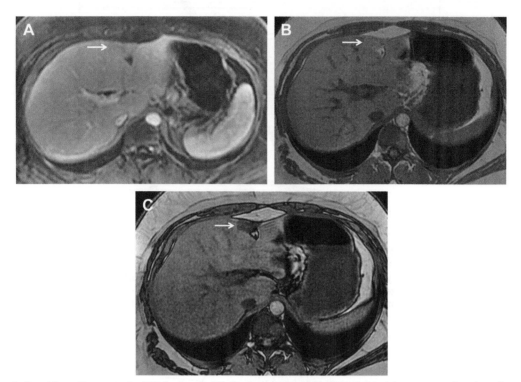

Fig. 6. Focal hepatic steatosis: MR features. (*A*) Contrast-enhanced T1-weighted image reveals a hypointense lesion (*arrow*) adjacent to the falciform ligament in the medial segment of the left lobe. (*B*) In-phase image shows that this lesion has mild hyperintensity (*arrow*). (*C*) Opposed-phase image shows that this region (*arrow*) loses significant signal intensity, indicating that this represents a focal area of fat deposition.

as adenomas (HA) and hepatocellular carcinomas (HCC).[47–51]

Hepatic Lipomas

Benign hepatic tumors composed of fat cells include lipoma, hibernoma, and combined tumors such as myelolipoma (fat and hematopoietic tissue), angiomyolipoma (fat and blood vessels), and angiomyelolipoma.[21]

Sonographically these lesions are highly echogenic and may be indistinguishable from HH.[45] On CT, these fatty tumors appear as well-defined masses with attenuation values in the range of fat (Fig. 11). Lipomas show high signal intensity on T1-weighted sequences and low signal intensity with fat-suppressed techniques. Lipomas show negligible enhancement following the administration of contrast material. Angiomyolipomas may not have a predominantly lipid content,

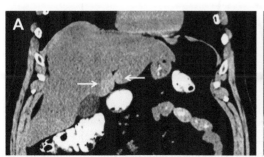
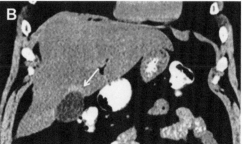

Fig. 7. Focal sparing in an otherwise fatty liver: CT findings. (*A*) Coronal reformatted image of the liver shows focal sparing from fatty infiltration in the medial and lateral segments of the left lobe (*arrows*). (*B*) Coronal reformatted image in the same patient shows sparing of fat deposition in the hepatic parenchyma adjacent to the gallbladder fossa (*arrows*).

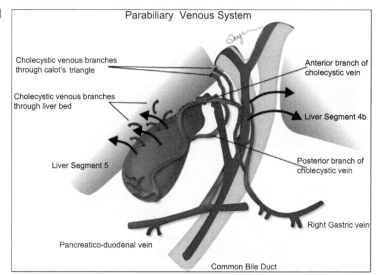

Fig. 8. Parabiliary venous system. These veins drain the gallbladder, stomach, and pancreatic head, and may connect to the main portal vein or drain directly into liver parenchyma (*black arrows*). These vessels are responsible for the presence of fatty deposition, fatty sparing, and THIDs (transient hepatic intensity differences) and THADs (transient hepatic attenuation differences) adjacent to the gallbladder fossa. (*From* Desser TS. Understanding transient hepatic attenuation differences. Semin Ultrasound CT MR 2009;30:408–17, Figure 4; with permission.)

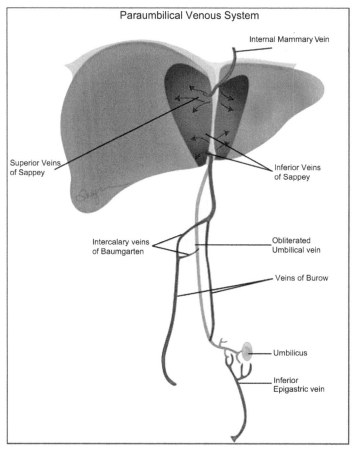

Fig. 9. The paraumbilical venous system. This system connects abdominal and chest wall vasculature to the inferior vena cava via collateral pathways that traverse the liver along its embryologic mesenteries (falciform ligament). These vessels account for the presence of fatty deposition, fatty sparing, and THIDs and THADs adjacent to the falciform ligament. (*From* Desser TS. Understanding transient hepatic attenuation differences. Semin Ultrasound CT MR 2009;30:408–17, Figure 3; with permission.)

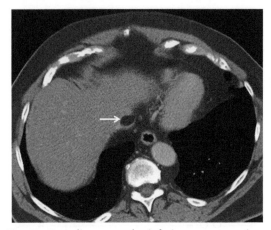

Fig. 10. Fat adjacent to the inferior vena cava simulating a caval tumor. Contrast-enhanced CT scan shows a fat density "mass" abutting the anterior aspect of the inferior vena cava (*arrow*). This variant is more commonly seen in patients with cirrhosis caused by the changes in hepatic morphology that accompany this disease.

Box 2
Flash-filling hepatic lesions
Hemangiomas
Focal nodular hyperplasia
THIDs
THADs
Adenomas
Nodular regenerative hyperplasia
Hypervascular metastases
Hepatocellular carcinoma
Fibrolamellar carcinoma
Arteriovenous malformations
Peliosis
Arterioportal shunts
Arteriovenous shunts
Portovenous shunts

and have a more complex pattern on MR that may be difficult to differentiate from HCC.[26,39]

HYPERVASCULAR FLASH-FILLING INCIDENTALOMAS

Small hypervascular, flash-filling hepatic defects are commonly found incidentally on MDCT. The differential diagnosis of these lesions is extensive and most are usually benign in patients with no history of malignancy, hepatic dysfunction, or hepatic risk factors. These lesions are listed in **Box 2** and discussed more fully in this section. Their imaging features are described in **Table 1**.

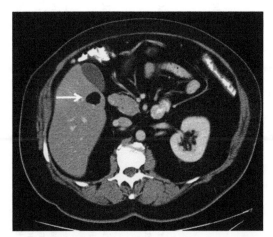

Fig. 11. Hepatic lipoma. Contrast-enhanced CT shows a well-marginated fat density (−58 HU) mass (*arrow*) in the right lobe of the liver.

Hepatic Hemangiomas

HHs are the most common benign tumor of the liver, with a reported incidence ranging from 1% to 20%.[21,52–54] These lesions are most commonly seen in women with a female/male ratio of 5:1.[21] In most cases, HHs are found incidentally on cross-sectional imaging examinations performed for symptoms and signs unrelated to this lesion. Most patients with HHs are asymptomatic and require no treatment. Clinical examination and laboratory tests are typically normal.[52,54]

HHs are composed of dilated endothelial-lined vascular channels, infiltrated by varying degrees of fibrous stroma. On cut sections, they appear spongy and are filled with dark venous blood. HHs are composed of varying-sized vascular channels, lined by a flattened endothelium underlined by a basement membrane, and separated by strands of fibrous stroma of various thicknesses. The vascular lumina are empty or blood-filled. Thrombi are frequent. According to the classic description, the interface between HH and the surrounding liver is well circumscribed and demarcated. However, there is generally no fibrous capsule and occasionally vascular channels may extend into the adjacent liver parenchyma.[20,21]

There are several variant types of HHs seen on cross-sectional imaging including: small (<2 cm) "flash-filling" lesions, which tend to enhance homogenously during the HAP; giant HHs (variably defined as >4–10 cm in diameter) with central nonenhancing scars; atypical centrifugally filling HHs;

Table 1
Imaging features of hypervascular flash-filling hepatic incidentalomas

Diagnosis	HAP	PVP	Delayed	MR Imaging	Scar	Hints
Small hemangioma <2 cm	Hypervascular THID or THAD	HYPER; follows blood pool	HYPER; follows blood pool	T2 HYPER; light bulb		Flash fill; follows blood pool Common in young women
Large hemangioma 2–10 cm	Nodular peripheral discontinuous enhancement THID or THAD	Centripetal enhancement	Progressive fill-in	T2 HYPER; light bulb		
FNH	Hyper	HYPER to ISO	ISO	T1 ISO T2 ISO	Progressive enhancement T2 HYPER	May contain fat Stealth lesions May only see on HAP
Adenomas	Hypervascular	Variable	Variable	Signal drop-out opposed phase		May contain fat May have hemorrhage; hyperdense NCCT
NRH	Hypervascular	HYPER to ISO	ISO	T1 ISO T2 ISO	If present similar to FNH	Found in liver with altered venous system
HCC	Hyperneovascularity	Variable	Hypo-washout	T2 hyperintense Similar to spleen		May contain fat May contain hemorrhage Often invades portal and hepatic veins
FLC	Heterogeneously hypervascular	Heterogeneous	Variable	T1 HYPO to ISO T2 HYPER	T1 HYPO T2 HYPO Calcifications	No fat Heterogeneous enhancement Calcification of central scar
Hypervascular metastases	Hypervascular May see rim or target sign THID or THAD	ISO or HYPO	ISO or HYPO Peripheral washout	T2 HYPER Similar to spleen		
Arterioportal shunts AVM	Hypervascular	ISO	ISO	ISO on T1 and T2		Usually nonspherical May regress spontaneously

Abbreviations: FLC, fibrolamellar carcinoma; FNH, focal nodular hyperplasia; HAP, hepatic arterial phase; HCC, hepatocellular carcinoma; HYPER, hyperdense on imaging; HYPO, hypodense on imaging; ISO, isodense on imaging; NCCT, noncontrast CT; NRH, nodular regenerative hyperplasia; PVP, portal venous phase; THAD, transient hepatic attenuation difference; THID, transient hepatic intensity difference.

From Kamaya A, Maturen KE, Tye GA, et al. Hypervascular liver lesions. Semin Ultrasound CT MR 2009;30:387–407; with permission.

and hyalinized HHs (also called sclerosed or sclerosing HHs), which may show little enhancement or delayed peripheral enhancement.[20,53]

Most HHs are discovered sonographically (Fig. 12) during right upper quadrant ultrasonography performed to rule out cholelithiasis. These lesions typically are well circumscribed and hyperechoic to normal hepatic parenchyma. In the setting of hepatic steatosis or cirrhosis, however, they may appear hypoechoic. Although this lesion is hyperechoic, in many cases HHs will exhibit posterior acoustic enhancement because the dilated, fluid-filled sacs of blood do not attenuate sound. An atypical but not uncommon sonographic appearance of HHs is a lesion with an echogenic rim with an internal hypoechoic pattern.[25]

HHs only rarely demonstrate internal flow on Doppler interrogation, due to the multidirectionality and slow velocity of flow. Though not currently approved for clinical use in the United States, contrast-enhanced sonography plays an important role in confirming the nature of HHs in Europe and Asia. Both a flash-filling and nodular, peripheral, centripetal pattern of enhancement can be seen, identical to the patterns identified on contrast-enhanced MDCT and MR imaging.[55–57]

On unenhanced CT scans, HHs have low attenuation compared with adjacent normal hepatic parenchyma, and when small may be impossible to differentiate from cysts. The classic enhancement pattern of HHs on HAP imaging is highly characteristic: peripheral, nodular, discontinuous enhancement isodense with the aorta, with progressive centripetal fill-in on subsequent phases. On PVP images, the lesions may become uniformly hyperenhancing compared with the normal parenchyma, which generally persists into delayed phases. Histologic correlation indicates that smaller vascular spaces enhance more quickly, and the spectrum, from HAP hyperattenuating nodules to gradually enhancing "puddles," reflects the variety of internal architecture of HHs.[20,53,58]

Small lesions (Fig. 13) often enhance uniformly producing a so-called flash-filling appearance, whereas large lesions (6–10 cm) often show central regions that do not exhibit contrast enhancement. HHs can also cause arterioportal shunting, which can simulate metastatic disease. It is important to image HHs over multiple phases to identify the characteristic pattern of enhancement.[20,45,53]

On MR, HHs typically have moderately low signal intensity on T1-weighted images and demonstrate marked hyperintensity on T2-weighted images, which may contain regions of low signal intensity corresponding with zones of fibrosis. HHs maintain high signal intensity on longer TE (>120 milliseconds), T2-weighted sequences. The majority of small (<1.5 cm) lesions show uniform flash filling. Medium-sized lesions (1.5–5 cm) show peripheral nodular enhancement progressing centripetally to uniform enhancement (Fig. 14). Most large lesions (>5 cm) exhibit peripheral nodular enhancement while the central portion remains hypointense.[26,45,59,60]

Small HHs often show robust, uniform, flash filling (Fig. 15) and may be difficult to differentiate

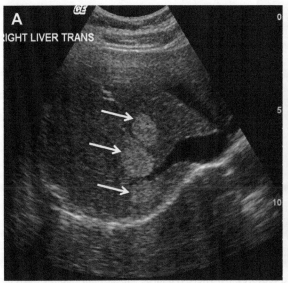
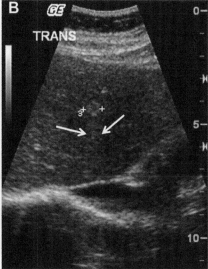

Fig. 12. Hepatic hemangiomas: sonographic features. (A) Axial sonogram shows 3 well-marginated, very echogenic hepatic lesions (arrows). (B) Sagittal sonogram shows a well-marginated mass (calipers) with acoustic enhancement (arrows), a sonographic hallmark of hepatic hemangiomas.

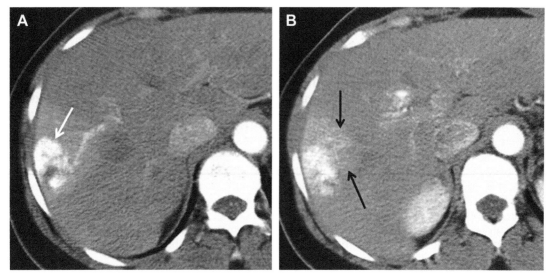

Fig. 13. Flash-filling hemangioma: CT features. Axial (*A* and *B*) contrast-enhanced CT images show a robustly enhancing hepatic mass (*white arrow*) associated with a prominent THAD (*black arrows*).

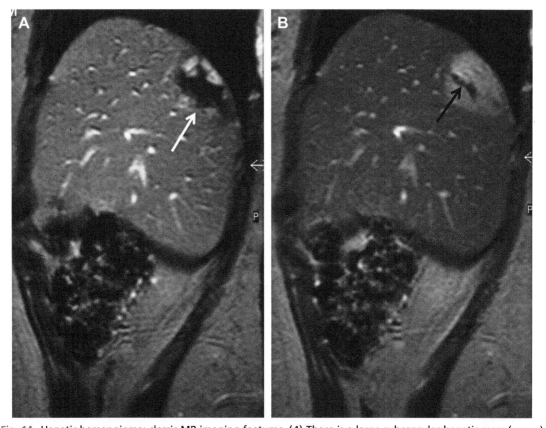

Fig. 14. Hepatic hemangioma: classic MR imaging features. (*A*) There is a large subcapsular hepatic mass (*arrow*) that shows peripheral nodular enhancement on this sagittal contrast-enhanced image. (*B*) Delayed sagittal image shows centripetal "filling in" of this mass, with the enhanced portions of the mass remaining isodense with the blood pool. Note the central scar (*arrow*) does not enhance.

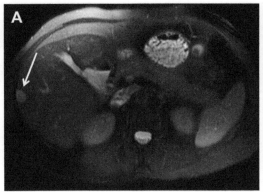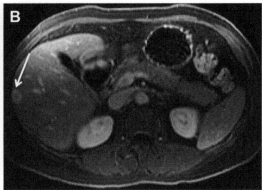

Fig. 15. Flash-filling hemangioma: MR imaging features. (*A*) Axial T2-weighted image shows a homogeneous, hyperintense hepatic lesion (*arrow*). (*B*) T1-weighted contrast-enhanced axial image demonstrates robust, homogeneous enhancement of this mass (*arrow*).

from other HAP enhancing neoplasms, such as HCC or hypervascular metastases. Distinguishing features, however, can be found on PVP and delayed images. Hypervascular neoplasms often show washout, whereas HHs show persistent enhancement.

Focal Nodular Hyperplasia

Focal nodular hyperplasia (FNH) is the second most common benign hepatic neoplasm, constituting 8% of primary hepatic tumors with an estimated prevalence of 0.9% and an 8:1 female-to-male predominance. These lesions are typically found incidentally at cross-sectional imaging, at elective surgery, or at autopsy. FNHs are most frequently found in women during the third to fifth decade of life. Although these lesions tend to occur in the same population as hepatic adenomas (HA), the pathogenesis of FNH is not believed to be related to oral contraceptive use, although hormonal contraceptives can have a trophic effect. In 80% to 85% of cases, FNH presents as a solitary lesion, most often less than 5 cm in size.[20,21,60]

FNH is defined microscopically as a tumor like condition characterized by a central fibrous scar with surrounding nodules of hyperplastic hepatocytes and small bile ductules. There is intense bile duct proliferation with a surrounding inflammatory infiltrate. Kupffer cells are invariably present. The nodules lack normal central veins and portal tracts. The bile ductules seen in the central scar do not connect to the biliary tract. Blood vessels course through the tumor and are most abundant in the fibrous scar.[20,21,60]

Grossly, FNH is a well-circumscribed solitary (95%) lesion that is typically located on the surface of the liver. On cut section, the majority of these tumors have an obvious central scar. Although

the margin is sharp, there is no capsule. Hemorrhage and necrosis are rare, and most tumors are less than 5 cm in size. FNH is believed to be a hyperplastic response to increased arterial flow in the setting of a vascular malformation, either congenital or acquired.[20,21,60–62]

Sonographically, FNH is usually nearly isoechoic and less commonly hypoechoic, with the normal liver parenchyma. Its contours are typically lobulated and a hypoechoic halo may occasionally be seen, producing a pseudocapsule appearance. A central stellate scar may be identified as a mildly hyperechoic structure in 20% of cases, particularly if the lesion is large.

On color Doppler sonography (Fig. 16), FNH shows increased blood flow, and a pattern of blood vessels radiating peripherally from a central feeding artery with a characteristic spoke-wheel pattern. Spectral Doppler analysis typically reveals a pulsatile, low-resistance waveform; occasionally, large peripheral draining veins may be seen. Contrast-enhanced ultrasonography demonstrates

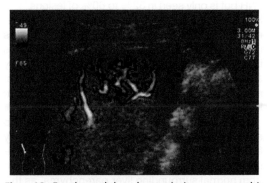

Fig. 16. Focal nodular hyperplasia: sonographic features. Color Doppler sonography shows increased blood flow and a spoke-wheel pattern of blood vessels radiating peripherally from a central feeding artery. Note the dilated feeding artery.

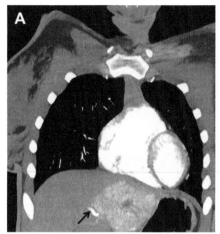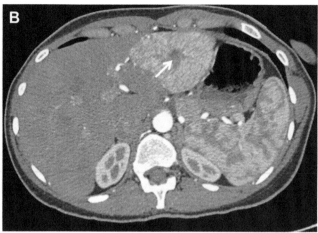

Fig. 17. Focal nodular hyperplasia: CT findings. Coronal (*A*) and axial (*B*) images performed during a pulmonary embolism study show a large incidental hypervascular hepatic mass with a central scar. Note the hypertrophied feeding artery and early draining vein (*black arrow*). The white arrow indicates the central scar.

early HAP enhancement with a centrifugal filling pattern, with the lesion becoming hyperechoic during the late HAP and slightly hyperechoic or isoechoic on the PVP and delayed phases.[25,63]

On nonenhanced CT scans, FNH usually appears as a homogeneous hypo- or isodense mass. In one-third of cases, a low-density central scar is visualized. During the HAP, FNH shows intense enhancement and the central scar remains hypodense (Fig. 17). During PVP, the difference in attenuation between FNH and normal liver promptly diminishes so that the tumor may be slightly hyperdense or isodense, with a hypo- or isodense central scar. On delayed imaging the lesion is isodense, but the central scar typically becomes hyperdense.[20,53,64]

Calcifications in the central scar are exceedingly rare and if present, fibrolamellar carcinoma (FLC) should be strongly considered. Though nonspecific, the central scar is a helpful distinguishing feature of FNH but is only seen in 32% to 60% of lesions.[65–67] FNH can be confidently diagnosed when a homogeneously and robustly enhancing, noncalcified mass is seen during HAP imaging that gradually becomes isodense on delayed images accompanied by a central scar, which slowly accretes contrast media. This classic appearance is most reliable in lesions larger than 3 cm.[68–72]

MR imaging has a higher sensitivity (70%) and specificity (98%) than MDCT and ultrasonography for the characterization of FNH.[73] On nonenhanced studies, FNH is often difficult to distinguish from normal surrounding liver parenchyma, as this tumor is isointense on T1-weighted images, and becomes slightly hyperintense to isointense on T2-weighted images. As with CT, the mass is characteristically homogeneous. The central scar is

hypointense on T1-weighted images and markedly hyperintense on T2-weighted images (Fig. 18), the latter being a distinguishing feature. MR visualizes the central scar in 78% of lesions.[74–76]

FNH enhances robustly and homogeneously during the HAP, with the exception of the late-enhancing central scar (Fig. 19). On both PVP and delayed imaging, the mass again becomes isointense or slightly hyperintense to the surrounding liver, with delayed enhancement of the central scar.[74–76]

The accurate diagnosis of FNHs is important because they are benign lesions with no risk of

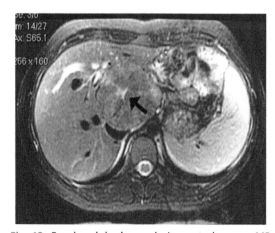

Fig. 18. Focal nodular hyperplasia: central scar on MR imaging. Axial unenhanced T2-weighted image shows a hyperintense central scar (*arrow*), a diagnostic finding in this lesion. (*From* Ros PR, Erturk SM. Benign tumors of the liver. In: Gore RM, Levine MS, editors. Textbook of gastrointestinal radiology. 3rd edition. Philadelphia: Saunders; 2008. p. 1603, Figure 88–13A; with permission.)

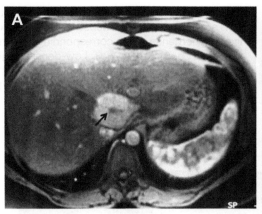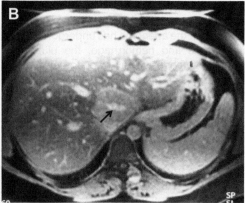

Fig. 19. Focal nodular hyperplasia: MR imaging features. (*A*) Arterial-phase axial T1-weighted image shows a robustly enhancing hepatic mass with the exception of the central scar (*arrow*). (*B*) Hepatic venous-phase axial T1-weighted image shows delayed enhancement of the central scar (*arrow*) while the remainder of the lesion is nearly isointense with normal hepatic parenchyma.

malignant degeneration, rupture, or hemorrhage. Several typical imaging characteristics of FNH can permit a confident diagnosis, including lesion homogeneity, delayed enhancement of a central scar, marked T2 hyperintensity of the central scar, homogeneous HAP enhancement, and the lack of a capsule. Although none of these features are specific when seen alone, the combination of several of them is suggestive.[20,53,64]

Hepatic Adenomas

Hepatocellular adenomas (HA) are rare, histologically benign neoplasms that have a small risk for malignant transformation into HCC, as well as a propensity for hemorrhage and rupture. The majority of these lesions occur in young women taking oral contraceptives. The estimated annual incidence in individuals with no history of oral contraceptive use is 1 in 1 million, which increases to 30 to 40 in 1 million with prolonged oral contraceptive use.[22] The risk of developing HAs is related to the both the duration of use and dose of hormones. The decline in the overall amount of hormones found in oral contraceptives has been paralleled by a decreased incidence of this tumor. These lesions regress when oral contraceptives are discontinued.[22]

Patients using estrogen- or androgen-containing medications are also at increased risk for HA development. Other populations noted to have an increased incidence of HAs include individuals with type I glycogen storage disease. In these patients, hepatic adenomas tend to be multiple.[20,22]

The classic clinical presentation of HAs is that of a spontaneous hemorrhage or rupture causing acute abdominal pain; however, most of the tumors are asymptomatic and found incidentally. In 70% to 80% of cases, HAs present as solitary lesions ranging in size from less than 1 cm to 15 cm. On gross pathology, adenomas are well-circumscribed, pale-yellow tumors that usually do not have a capsule. Histologically, they are composed of sheets of cells resembling normal hepatocytes containing abundant glycogen and lipid. Prominent arteries and draining veins are seen; however, the tumor lacks portal tracts and terminal hepatic veins. Kupffer cells are present in up to 20% of cases. Fatty hepatocytes are frequently present.[21,22]

The imaging features of HAs depend on the amount of lipid, hemorrhage, or fibrosis within the tumor, and the status of the surrounding hepatic parenchyma.

The sonographic findings (**Fig. 20**) are usually variable and nonspecific, but HAs typically

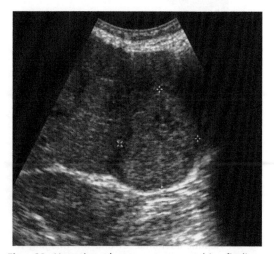

Fig. 20. Hepatic adenoma: sonographic findings. Sagittal sonogram reveals a nonspecific appearing echogenic mass (calipers) with a hypoechoic region centrally corresponding to an area of hemorrhage.

manifest as a large hyperechoic lesion with central anechoic areas, corresponding to zones of internal hemorrhage. If the adenoma has undergone significant necrosis and hemorrhage, the ultrasonographic appearance is that of a complex mass with large cystic components. Color Doppler evaluation can be helpful, demonstrating peripheral and intratumoral vessels showing a flat continuous Doppler waveform in contrast to the usual pulsatile waveform of FNH and HCC.[25,77,78]

On unenhanced CT (Fig. 21A), uncomplicated HAs are isodense or hypodense to the surrounding liver. Hyperdense areas corresponding to hemorrhage can be noted as well. Low-density regions may correspond to regions of intratumoral fat.

Following contrast administration, CT (see Fig. 21B, C) shows homogeneous enhancement on HAP imaging in 81% to 90% of cases, particularly if the lesions are small (<3 cm). The enhancement is moderate and remains less than that of the

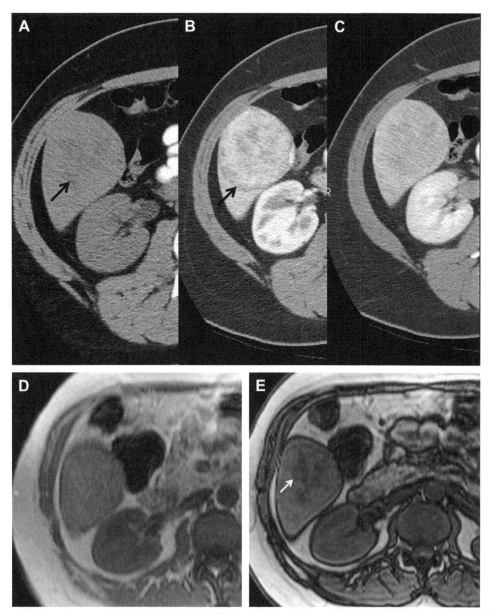

Fig. 21. Hepatic adenoma: CT and MR imaging features. (A) Axial unenhanced CT scan shows a low-density hepatic mass (*black arrows*) with focal areas of fat. This lesion exhibits moderate, inhomogeneous contrast enhancement on hepatic arterial phase image (B) that shows gradual washout on delayed phase (C) CT image. In-phase (D) and opposed-phase (E) MR images reveal drop-out of signal intensity by the fat within this tumor (*white arrow*).

arterial vasculature. It is less impressive and more heterogeneous than seen in FNH. On PVP and delayed imaging, the lesion is nearly isodense to the surrounding liver. Due to the presence of necrosis, fat, and hemorrhage, some 25% of lesions will have a more heterogeneous appearance. Fat has been identified in 7% of lesions and calcifications are present in 5% to 15%. Larger lesions tend to be more heterogeneous than smaller lesions, and the CT appearance is nonspecific.[53,79]

HAs do not have a central scar, a point useful in distinguishing the lesion from FNH, which tends to occur in the same patient population. In the background of hepatic steatosis, HAs typically are hyperdense on all phases.[78,79]

By virtue of its ability to depict internal lipid content (see **Fig. 21**D, E) and hemorrhage with in- and opposed-phase sequences and superior contrast resolution, MR imaging can often better characterize HAs.[26]

HAs can be isointense on T1-weighted sequences or may be hyperintense due to fat content. HAs are quite variable in T2 signal intensity and often show signal dropout on opposed-phase imaging (**Fig. 22**). Following gadolinium administration, there is faint enhancement during the HAP only, with an isointense appearance on delayed imaging. A peripheral rim can be seen in up to one-third of lesions, representing the variably present fibrous capsule. Unlike FNH lesions, HAs do not take up superparamagnetic iron oxide particles because they lack Kupffer cells. Similarly, there is no significant uptake of hepatocellular-specific contrast agents by HAs. Scintigraphic studies are not particularly useful for HA characterization, as they do not demonstrate uptake on either Tc-99m sulfur colloid scans or iminodiacetic acid studies.[80,81]

Although benign, HAs are important to accurately diagnose, because 10% of patients will present acutely due to adenoma rupture and subsequent hemoperitoneum. Furthermore, there is a risk of malignant degeneration in up to 10% of tumors. Both of these risks are more pronounced with larger lesions. For these reasons, HAs are typically surgically resected. Although the characteristics of the mass on CT and/or MR can often result in a confident diagnosis, there is still occasional overlap between the appearance of an adenoma and that of FNH, which also occurs in young women. Brancatelli and colleagues[81] have noted that in these cases, the most useful distinguishing features are the presence or absence of a central scar as well as the signal characteristics on MR indicating the presence or absence of fat and the degree of lesion heterogeneity. Furthermore, a well-differentiated HCC can have many of the same imaging features as those of an HA and in these cases, clinical correlation with other features, such as the presence of cirrhosis and the patient's serum α-fetoprotein, may be helpful in narrowing the differential diagnosis.[81]

Nodular Regenerative Hyperplasia

Nodular regenerative hyperplasia (NRH) is defined as a diffuse nodularity of the liver produced by

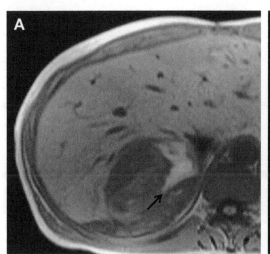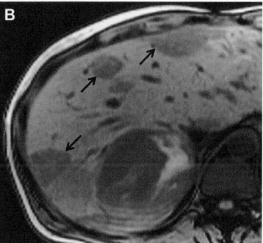

Fig. 22. Intralesional fat and hemorrhage in a patient with multiple hepatic adenomas. (*A*) In-phase axial MR image shows a large low-signal mass that contains regions of high signal intensity, indicating intralesional hemorrhage (*arrow*). (*B*) Opposed-phase axial MR image demonstrates additional lesions (*arrows*) with low signal intensity due intratumoral fat. The hemorrhagic mass also shows loss of signal intensity, indicating the presence of fat.

many regenerative nodules that are not associated with fibrosis.[20,39,82] NRH grossly is characterized by the presence of multiple bulging subcapsular nodules that on cut surface appear as discrete, round, flat nodules that resemble diffuse involvement with metastatic carcinoma. These nodules vary in size from a few millimeters to several centimeters and are diffusely scattered. Microscopically, the nodules are composed of cells resembling normal hepatocytes, and no fibrosis is noted; this is an important difference between NRH and regenerating nodules of cirrhosis.[21,39,82]

NRH is rare, although some autopsy series have shown a prevalence as high as 0.6%.[21] NRH is associated with various systemic disease and drugs that are also associated with the Budd-Chiari syndrome: polycythemia vera, chronic myelogenous leukemia, myeloid metaplasia, Hodgkin disease and non-Hodgkin lymphoma, chronic lymphocytic leukemia, rheumatoid arthritis, Felty syndrome, polyarteritis nodosa, scleroderma, systemic lupus erythematosis, steroids, and antineoplastic medications.[21,39,82]

The sonographic appearance of NRH is variable, ranging from normal to a liver with multiple focal nodules that vary in echogenicity. Central hemorrhage with a large nodule may occur and produce a complex mass.[25,83] The CT appearance of NRH is also variable. On unenhanced scans, these lesions are usually hypodense but when hemorrhagic, they may produce a complex mass with variable density. On contrast-enhanced scans, HAP imaging shows hypervascular lesions (Fig. 23) that may become almost imperceptible during the PVP. On unenhanced MR imaging, NRH lesions are usually isointense to normal liver on T2-weighted images and contain foci of high signal on T1-weighted scans. As on CT, these lesions often show robust contrast enhancement.[84]

Hepatocellular Carcinoma

HCC is the third leading cause of cancer-related death worldwide, and risk factors include hepatitis B carrier state, chronic hepatitis C virus infection, hemochromatosis, exposure to aflatoxins, and cirrhosis from any cause. Nonalcoholic steatohepatitis is a recently recognized risk factor that, in view of the obesity epidemic in the United States, has the potential to make this disorder a major risk factor for HCC. There are significant geographic factors in HCC incidence, reflecting the heterogeneous distribution of its main etiologic factors. Usually the diagnosis is made in symptomatic patients, in patients with known cirrhosis, or in those undergoing screening and surveillance examinations.[21,85–89]

In cirrhotic patients it is important to distinguish early small HCCs from macroregenerative nodules and dysplastic nodules, as well as atypical hemangiomas and metastases.

HCC has a varied, nonspecific appearance on ultrasonography. Small HCCs (<3 cm) often appear hypoechoic (Fig. 24) but may be hyperechoic,

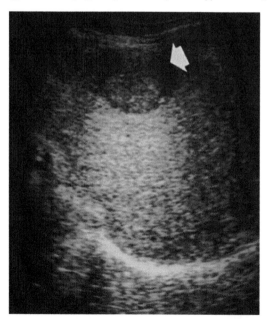

Fig. 24. Hepatocellular carcinoma: sonographic features. Sonogram demonstrates a hypoechoic mass with a peripheral halo sign (*arrow*). (*From* Ros PR, Erturk SM. Malignant tumors of the liver. In: Gore RM, Levine MS, editors. Textbook of gastrointestinal radiology. 3rd edition. Philadelphia: Saunders; 2008, p. 1627, Figure 89–4E; with permission.)

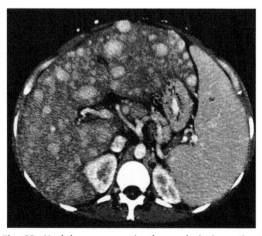

Fig. 23. Nodular regenerative hyperplasia in patient with Budd-Chiari syndrome: imaging features. Axial contrast enhance CT scan shows multiple hyperenhancing hepatic masses. (Case *Courtesy of* Michael P. Federle, MD and Richard L. Baron, MD.)

particularly if there is fatty change or marked sinusoidal dilatation. Tumors larger than 3 cm more often have a mosaic or mixed pattern. The capsule of encapsulated HCCs may appear as a thin, hypoechoic band.[21,85,90–92]

On unenhanced CT scans, HCCs may present as hypodense lesions, due to necrosis and/or the presence of fat. Because these neoplasms derive the majority of their blood supply from the hepatic artery, they demonstrate robust enhancement during the HAP and are relatively hypodense on the delayed-phase images (Fig. 25). The tumor has a variable appearance on PVP images, including isodense with the remainder of the liver. The capsule appears either isodense or hypodense relative to the liver during the HAP and enhances on delayed CT images.[85,93–96]

HCC has a variable appearance on MR imaging. It shows intermediate to high signal intensity on T2-weighted images, similar in intensity to the spleen, and variable intensity on T1-weighted images, depending on the presence of internal fibrosis, fatty change, and the dominant histologic pattern.[26,53,97,98]

As with CT, HCC shows robust enhancement during the HAP phase. These vascular lesions often show contrast washout to a greater degree than the adjacent hepatic parenchyma (Fig. 26). The washout phenomenon can help differentiate HCCs from other hypervascular lesions.[53,85]

When well differentiated, HCCs may not be hypervascular on HAP images. However, if a well-defined capsule and internal washout are demonstrated on delayed-phase images, the diagnosis can be suggested. Larger lesions often have areas of neovascularity and central areas of necrosis if they outgrow their blood supply. HCCs may occasionally contain areas of fat and may spontaneously bleed, especially when exophytic.[53]

Fibrolamellar Carcinoma

Fibrolamellar carcinoma (FLC) is a slow-growing hepatic neoplasm that arises in a normal liver. FLC is composed of neoplastic hepatocytes separated into cords by lamellar fibrous strands. The most common variant of FLC shows areas of glandular-type differentiation with mucin production. FLC does not commonly cause elevation of α-fetoprotein, and no reliable serum tumor markers have been identified.[22] This tumor usually occurs in adolescents and adults younger than 40 years without predisposing risk factors. When symptomatic, patients may present with pain, malaise, weight loss, and occasionally jaundice.[20]

At presentation, FLC is generally a large, solitary mass, usually 5 to 20 cm in size, with well-defined and lobulated margins. Small peripheral satellite lesions may, on occasion, be present. FLCs often have an irregular central scar (seen in 20%–71% of patients) and coarse calcifications within the central scar (seen in 35%–68% of patients).[99,100]

Sonographically, FLCs usually present as a large, well-defined, lobulated mass with mixed echogenicity. A central scar may be visualized as a central area of hyperechogenicity.[25,99,100]

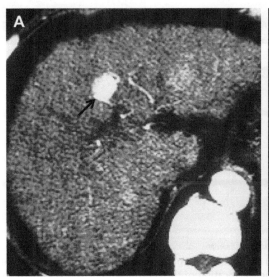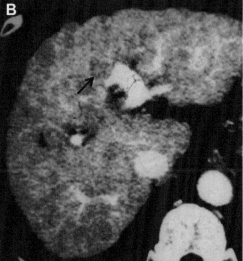

Fig. 25. Hepatocellular carcinoma: CT findings. (A) Axial CT scan obtained from a patient with cirrhosis during the hepatic arterial phase demonstrates a small flash-filling mass (arrow) in the medial segment of the left lobe. (B) This mass becomes hypodense (arrow) on portal venous phase images.

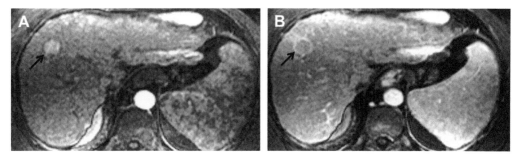

Fig. 26. Hepatocellular carcinoma: MR findings. Axial enhanced scans show a robustly enhancing tumor (*arrow*) during the arterial phase (*A*), which demonstrates washout with ring enhancement on the portal venous phase image (*arrow*) (*B*). (*From* Ros PR, Erturk SM. Malignant tumors of the liver. In: Gore RM, Levine MS, editors. Textbook of gastrointestinal radiology. 3rd edition. Philadelphia: Saunders; 2008. p. 1631, Figures 89–9 E and F; with permission.)

On unenhanced CT scans, FLC appears as a hypodense mass with a well-defined contour. Stellate calcifications may be found within the central scar (Fig. 27A). On contrast-enhanced CT, FLCs are typically heterogeneously hypervascular with avidly enhancing tumor vessels. Enhancement on PVP and delayed-phase images is variable, which reflects washout of the contrast from more vascular areas of the tumor together with delayed enhancement of the fibrous lamellae. The central scar is generally low on both pre- and postcontrast CT but may show delayed enhancement, simulating FNH.[85,101,102]

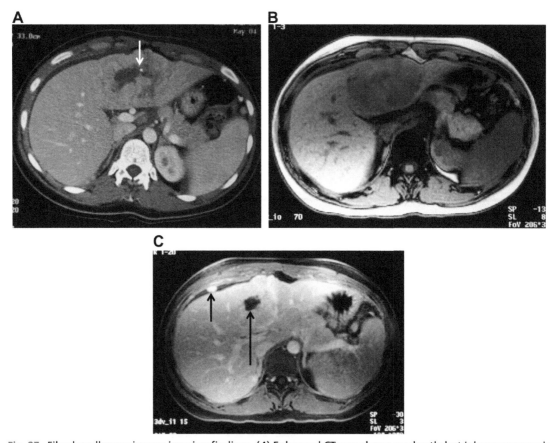

Fig. 27. Fibrolamellar carcinoma: imaging findings. (*A*) Enhanced CT scan shows a robustly but inhomogeneously enhancing lesion in the left lobe of the liver. Notice the calcification of the central scar (*arrow*). (*B*) Unenhanced T1-weighted MR scan in the same patient shows an inhomogeneous, low signal-intensity mass. (*C*) Following contrast administration, this mass (*large arrow*) shows robust enhancement except for the scar. There is ascites and an enhancing peritoneal metastasis (*small arrow*).

On MR imaging (see **Fig. 27**B, C), FLCs are generally hypo- to isointense relative to normal hepatic parenchyma on T1-weighted images, and slightly hyperintense on T2-weighted sequences. Because of its purely fibrous nature, the central scar is hypointense on T1- and T2-weighted images, a differentiating feature from FNH. In addition, the central scar shows minimal or no enhancement. Hypointense septa radiating toward the tumor periphery may be better appreciated on MR imaging than on CT. FLCs have no detectable intrinsic fat.[26,53,103]

The major differential diagnosis of FLC is FNH because both occur in the same age group. Differentiating features include: the central scar of FNH is hyperintense on T2-weighted images; FNH only rarely calcifies (<1.5% of cases compared with up to 55% of FLCs); and FNH is usually asymptomatic whereas patients with FLC typically present with symptoms.[53]

Hypervascular Metastases

Metastases are the most common malignant liver tumors, and occur 20 times more frequently than primary hepatic neoplasms. The liver is second only to regional lymph nodes as a site of metastatic disease, and approximately 25% to 50% of all patients who die of cancer have liver metastases at autopsy.[22,104] Except for infiltrative tumors such as lymphoma, most metastases manifest as multiple discrete lesions. The imaging appearance of metastases can vary greatly depending on differences or blood supply, hemorrhage, cellular differentiation, fibrosis, and necrosis.

Most liver metastases are hypovascular, and as a result are hypointense on MR imaging and hypodense on CT as compared with normal liver parenchyma during the PVP. Colon, lung, breast, and gastric cancers are the most common causes of hypovascular liver metastases. These metastases are best visualized during the PVP and typically showing perilesional enhancement or a target appearance. If the lesions do not show this appearance, small hypodense or hypointense metastases may be difficult to differentiate from a host of benign hepatic lesions described earlier.[53,105]

Hypervascular metastases enhance earlier and are most conspicuous on the HAP. In addition, they demonstrate variable degrees of washout on delayed images. The most common causes of hypervascular hepatic metastases include neuroendocrine tumors (eg, carcinoid, pheochromocytoma, and islet cell tumors), renal cell carcinoma, melanoma, choriocarcinoma, and thyroid carcinoma. Breast carcinoma and, rarely, pancreatic adenocarcinoma can also cause hypervascular metastases.[53,105]

Hypervascular metastases smaller than 1.5 cm can be difficult to distinguish from flash-filling HHs, because both can display rapid enhancement during HAP contrast-enhanced CT and MR imaging (**Figs. 28** and **29**) and increased T2 signal intensity on MR imaging. On PVP or delayed-phase imaging, however, they do have a distinctly different appearance. HHs retain their contrast material and appear enhanced during the PVP, whereas hypervascular metastases tend to wash out. Another potential distinguishing feature is

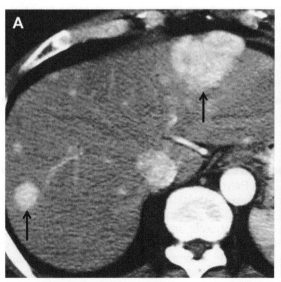
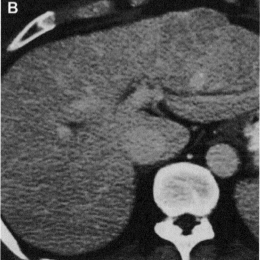

Fig. 28. Hypervascular liver metastases: CT features. (*A*) Arterial-phase scan shows multiple flash filling hepatic masses (*arrows*). These lesions show prompt washout during the portal venous phase (*B*).

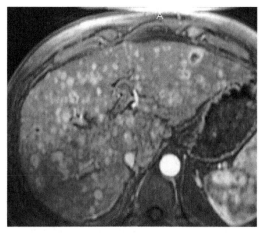

Fig. 29. Hypervascular metastases: MR features. Multiple enhancing hepatic masses are identified on this contrast-enhanced axial MR scan in a patient with metastatic renal cell carcinoma.

the "peripheral washout" sign, a specific but insensitive sign for malignancy that favors the diagnosis of metastasis or HCC over HH. Malignant lesions often show peripheral washout of contrast on delayed contrast-enhanced images, and a target appearance, with the rim appearing hypointense relative to the center. This target appearance has been reported to be highly specific for hypervascular metastasis (100% specificity) and is frequently observed in hypervascular metastases from neuroendocrine and carcinoid tumors.[105,106]

Transient Hepatic Attenuation Differences and Transient Hepatic Intensity Differences

Intrahepatic parenchymal perfusion disorders such as THIDs and THADs are epiphenomena of alterations of the dual vascular supply of the liver seen on MR and CT, respectively. There is a compensatory relationship between hepatic arterial and portal venous blood supply so that arterial flow increases when portal blood flow decreases. This situation is made possible by communication among the main vessels, sinusoids, and peribiliary venules that dilate in response to autonomic nervous activity and humoral factors activated by hepatic demand for oxygen and metabolites. THADs and THIDs are areas of parenchymal enhancement on CT and MR visible during the HAP following the intravenous administration of contrast material. These "lesions" are an increasingly common cause of hepatic incidentalomas, and can be classified by morphology, etiology, and pathogenesis.[43,107–128]

THADs and THIDs associated with a true hepatic mass

Malignant and benign (Fig. 30) hepatic masses produce 2 morphologic types of THIDs and THADs via 4 major pathophysiologic mechanisms: direct siphoning effect of the mass (lobar multisegmental shape), or indirectly by means of portal hypoperfusion (sectorial shape) due to portal branch compression or infiltration, by thrombus resulting in a portal branch blockade, or by flow diversion caused by an arterioportal shunt.[43,107–111,113–128]

Lobar multisegmental THADs and THIDs occur when a benign hypervascular lesion or an abscess induces an increase in the primary arterial inflow, which leads to surrounding parenchymal perfusion, the so-called siphoning effect. These THADs and THIDs do not assume a triangular shape, but a straight border may be present between the arterial phenomenon and the "normal" adjacent parenchyma.[43,107–111,113–128]

Sectorial THADs and THIDs follow hepatic vessel dichotomy and appear as triangular areas that result from the strict relationship between the portal hypoperfused area and the arterial reaction. These lesions can be seen in benign and malignant tumors as well as abscesses caused by the spread of inflammatory mediators. The THADs and THIDs can be wedge- or fan-shaped in this instance.[43,107–111,113–128]

THADs and THIDs not associated with a mass lesion

THIDs and THADs can be seen in the absence of a focal lesion as a result of 3 mechanisms: portal hypoperfusion due to portal branch compression or thrombosis (Fig. 31); flow diversion by arterioportal shunts or by an anomalous blood supply; or inflammation or obstruction of the bile ducts or gallbladder.[43,107–111,113–128]

Sectorial THADs and THIDs are usually caused by portal hypoperfusion caused by portal vein or hepatic vein thrombosis, long-standing biliary obstruction, or an arterioportal shunt that may be congenital, traumatic, or caused by cirrhosis. These THADs and THIDs can have a globular shape, especially when they are adjacent to Glisson's capsule.[43,107–111,113–128]

Polymorphous THADs and THIDs have 4 major causes: external compression by a rib or subcapsular fluid collection; anomalous blood supply from atypical arteries, collateral venous vessels, or accessory veins, especially in segment IV of the liver; inflammation of adjacent organs such as cholecystitis and pancreatitis that spread inflammatory mediators and reduce portal inflow due to interstitial edema; and posttraumatic,

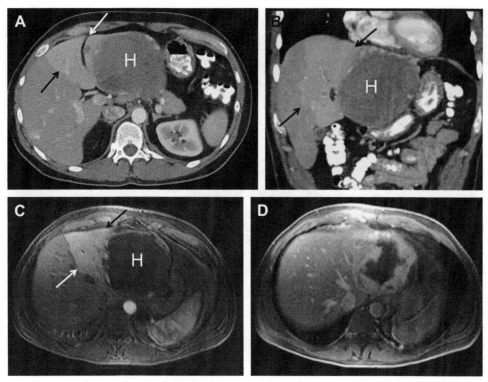

Fig. 30. THADs and THIDs associated with a benign mass: imaging features. Axial (*A*) and coronal (*B*) scans show a large hemangioma (H) in the lateral segment of the left lobe, causing a large THAD in the medial segment (*arrows*). Early (*C*) and late (*D*) phase MR images show a THID (H) on the early-phase images and resolution on the delayed scan, which also shows filling in of the hemangioma (H).

postbiopsy, postradiofrequency ablation of hepatic tumors.[43,107–111,113–128]

In patients with obstruction of the superior vena cava, the medial segment of the left lobe (segment IV) of the liver will often show hyperenhancement (**Fig. 32**) due to collateral veins. The internal mammary vein connects to the left portal vein via the paraumbilical vein. Diffuse THADs and THIDs can be seen in right-sided heart failure, the

Budd-Chiari syndrome, and biliary obstruction, leading to abnormal attenuation and signal intensity adjacent to the portal triads.[43,107–111,113–128]

Arteriovenous Malformations and Intrahepatic Vascular Shunts

Hepatic arteriovenous malformation (AVM) is congenital abnormality of blood vessels that

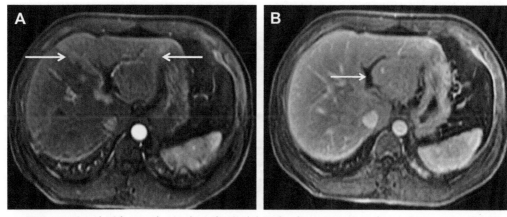

Fig. 31. THID associated with portal vein thrombosis. (*A*) Early-phase contrast-enhanced MR image shows clot in the ascending portion of the left portal vein producing a THID (*arrows*). On delayed images (*B*) the THID resolves. Arrow indicates thrombus.

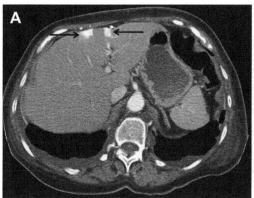
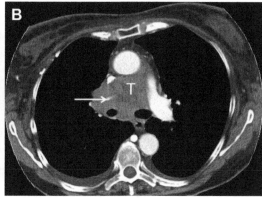

Fig. 32. THAD caused by superior vena cava obstruction by metastatic lung cancer. (*A*) Axial CT scan shows flash-filling lesions (*arrows*) along the anterior aspect of the medial segment of the left hepatic lobe. (*B*) Axial contrast-enhanced chest CT scan shows tumor (T) obstructing the superior vena cava (*arrow*).

results in the shunting of blood through direct communications between the arterial venous channels. These vascular anomalies contain no abnormal tissue between the anomalous vessels.[22,59,129,130]

Sonographically, hepatic AVMs appear as a cluster of enlarged, tortuous vessels confined to one lobe of the liver with increased venous pulsatility, decreased resistive indices, arterialization of portal flow, reversal of portal flow, and/or aliasing on color Doppler imaging due increased turbulence and flow velocity. The hepatic artery is frequently enlarged.[59,129,130]

AVMs show intense homogeneous enhancement on CT (**Fig. 33**) and MR during the HAP and early PVP images.

Three types of intrahepatic vascular shunting may occur: arterial to portal venous, arterial to hepatic venous, and portal to hepatic venous. Abnormal vascular connections between the hepatic arterial system and portal venous system can arise within hypervascular masses (eg, HCC, metastases), in the cirrhotic liver, secondary to

trauma (eg, biopsy), or rarely through rupture of hepatic artery aneurysms into the adjacent portal vein. The common pathophysiology of all arterioportal shunting involves the entry of arterial blood at systolic pressures into the low-pressure portal venous system; subsequently, localized reversal of portal flow occurs and local parenchyma is subjected to increased perfusion pressure. Altered and arterial dominant vascular supply to the localized parenchyma may cause a THAD, a THID, and/or focal fatty infiltration or sparing in a fatty liver, when small, intrahepatic vascular malformations may manifest as "color spots" on Doppler sonography.[59,129,130]

INCIDENTALOMAS IN SPECIFIC PATIENT COHORTS

Hepatic Incidentalomas in the Oncology Patient

When evaluating a small hepatic mass in the oncology patient, 2 important facts must be considered. First, at postmortem examination,

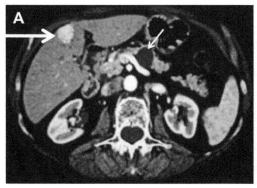
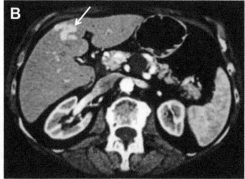

Fig. 33. Arteriovenous malformation: CT features. (*A*) Contrast-enhanced CT scan shows a hypervascular lesion (*large arrow*) in the left lobe of the liver and an incidental cystic pancreatic lesion (*small arrow*). (*B*) Scan obtained caudal to (*A*) shows a tortuous feeding artery (*arrow*). (Case *Courtesy of* Elliot K. Fishman, MD.)

benign hepatic lesions are detected in up to 52% of the general population.[20,22] Second, the liver is the most common site of extranodal metastases, seen in up to 36% of patients.[22] Small hepatic masses are commonly encountered in both populations on cross-sectional imaging. Hepatic cysts including BDHs and HHs are present in nearly 40% of patients.[22] When less than 1.5 cm in size, these lesions can be difficult to characterize and differentiate from metastatic disease.[131–135] Several studies have specifically addressed this issue.

Jones and colleagues[136] found at least one hepatic lesion 1.5 cm or smaller in 17% of all patients in a retrospective study performed on nonhelical CT scanners. In patients with a known malignancy, 51% were benign, 26% were malignant, and 23% were indeterminate. The likelihood of malignancy was 5% with 1 lesion, 19% with 2 to 4 lesions, and 74% with 5 or more lesions. In a second study of 2978 patients with cancer, Schwartz and colleagues[137] found small ($\leq$1.0 cm) lesions in 12.7% of patients, of which 80.2% were benign, 11.6% were malignant, and 8.2% were indeterminate.

Studies performed with helical scanners have also found the majority of small, low-attenuating lesions within the liver in the oncology patient to be benign. In a review of 1133 patients with colorectal and gastric cancer, Jang and colleagues[138] found small ($\leq$1.5 cm) hypoattenuating lesions in 25.5% of cases. Some 94% of lesions that were smooth and low density ($\leq$20 HU) proved to be benign. In a study of 941 women with breast cancer, Khalil and coworkers[139] found 1 or more small, hypoattenuating lesion in 29.4%. In 92.7% of patients these lesions showed no change, in 4.2% they disappeared, and in 3.1% they became larger. The investigators concluded that finding a small, hypodense lesion in the liver with no definite metastases was a benign finding. Krakora and colleagues,[140] in a study of 153 patients with breast cancer, discovered small hypoattenuating hepatic lesions in 35%, noting that the presence of these small lesions without definite hepatic metastases did not contribute an increased risk of developing subsequent hepatic metastases.

The imaging findings and differential diagnosis of hypervascular metastases are described in an earlier section.

Hepatic Incidentalomas in the Patient with Diffuse Hepatic Steatosis

Severe hepatic steatosis may alter the apparent enhancement pattern of focal hepatic lesions. Even hypovascular tumors such as metastases can show relatively high attenuation on CT and simulate

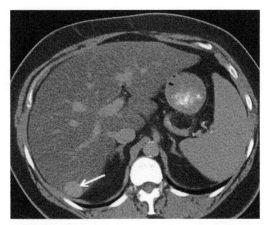

Fig. 34. Hemangioma in a fatty liver: CT findings. A small hyperdense lesion (*arrow*) is identified in the right lobe, which is isodense with the blood pool.

HHs with a persistent contrast enhancement pattern. On unenhanced scans, the density of an HH may appear hyperattenuating, though not greater than that of blood vessels (Fig. 34). HHs may also be accompanied by a focal spared zone as seen in malignant tumors in fatty liver. This finding can create confusion sonographically, with a hypoechoic halo surrounding the HH simulating that seen in malignant tumors rather than the usual hyperechoic rim surrounding the HH. This unusual finding often makes subsequent CT or MR imaging necessary. HHs in fatty liver can produce a peculiar halo on CT or MR imaging as well, but in most cases accurate diagnosis can be made without difficulty because of the characteristic dynamic enhancement pattern of HHs.

Focal hepatic steatosis is a common pseudotumor detected on ultrasonography, MDCT, and MR

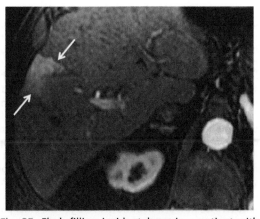

Fig. 35. Flash-filling incidentaloma in a patient with cirrhosis: MR findings. Contrast-enhanced axial scan shows a wedge-shaped hyperenhancing area (*arrow*) in the right lobe. Subsequent evaluation showed no underlying mass.

imaging that can be problematic in the oncology patient. On MDCT, focal fat appears as an area of decreased attenuation that does not cause mass effect and through which blood vessels normally course. If the diagnosis is uncertain, steatosis can be confirmed with in-phase and opposed-phase MR imaging, which is described

below. These pseudotumors are described more fully in an earlier section.

Hepatic Incidentalomas in the Patient with Cirrhosis

Small, peripheral, THIDs (Fig. 35) and THADs are commonly seen in the cirrhotic liver. These lesions

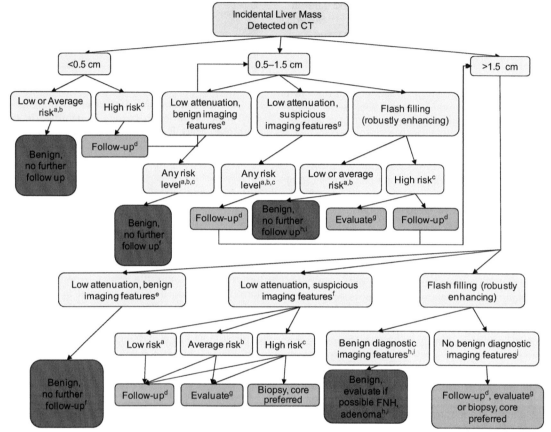

Fig. 36. Algorithm for the evaluation of the hepatic incidentaloma. [a] Low-risk individuals: young patient (≤40 years old), with no known malignancy, hepatic dysfunction, hepatic malignant risk factors, or symptoms attributable to the liver. [b] Average-risk individuals: patient >40 years old, with no known malignancy, hepatic dysfunction, or hepatic malignant risk factors or symptoms attributable to the liver. [c] High risk individuals: known primary malignancy with a propensity to metastasize to the liver, cirrhosis, and/or other hepatic risk factors. Hepatic risk factors include hepatitis, chronic active hepatitis, sclerosing cholangitis, primary biliary cirrhosis, hemochromatosis, hemosiderosis, oral contraceptive use, and anabolic steroid use. [d] Follow-up CT or MR imaging in 6 months. May need more frequent follow-up in some situations, for example, a cirrhotic patient who is a liver transplant candidate. [e] Benign imaging features: typical hemangioma (see below), sharply marginated, homogeneous low attenuation up to about 20 HU, no enhancement. May have sharp, but irregular shape. [f] Benign low-attenuation masses: cyst, hemangioma, hamartoma, von Meyenburg complex (bile duct hamartomas). [g] Suspicious imaging features: ill-defined margins, enhancement (more than about 20 HU), heterogeneous, enlargement. To evaluate, prefer multiphasic MR imaging. [h] Hemangioma features: nodular discontinuous peripheral enhancement with progressive enlargement of enhancing foci on subsequent phases. Nodule isodense with vessels, not parenchyma. [i] Small robustly enhancing lesion in average-risk, young patient: hemangioma, FNH, transient hepatic attenuation difference (THAD) flow artifact, and in average-risk, older patient: hemangioma, THAD flow artifact. Other possible diagnoses: adenoma, AVM, nodular regenerative hyperplasia. Differentiation of FNH from adenoma is important, especially if larger than 4 cm and subcapsular. [j] Hepatocellular or common metastatic enhancing malignancy: islet cell, neuroendocrine, carcinoid, renal cell carcinoma, melanoma, choriocarcinoma, sarcoma, breast, some pancreatic lesions. (*From* Berland LL, Silverman SG, Gore RM, et al. Managing incidental findings on abdominal CT: white paper of the ACR Incidental Finding Committee. J Am Coll Radiol 2010;7:754–73; with permission.)

probably arise from portal hypoperfusion in the context of portal hypertension and even occlusion, permitting focal arterial dominance and resulting in a hypervascular imaging appearance. These lesions are not true masses but rather represent foci of abnormal vascularity; they have no clinical significance except as a marker for underlying hepatocellular disease, but may simulate HCC and other hepatic tumors.[140,141]

During the HAP of enhancement on CT and MR imaging, peripheral subcentimeter nodular or irregular hypervascular foci denote the actual site of vascular connection. HAP images sometimes depict early intravascular enhancement of the associated portal vein branch. During the PVP, the hypervascular nodule becomes much less conspicuous or entirely undetectable. On follow-up imaging months to years later, most nontumorous arterioportal shunts in chronic liver disease disappear or spontaneously regress. The enhancement patterns in MR imaging are almost perfectly analogous to CT, but the lesions are not visible on precontrast T1- and T2-weighted imaging. The tiny foci of AP shunting in cirrhosis are not usually visible sonographically due to the hyperechogenicity and scarring of the liver. Indeed, most hypervascular lesions in cirrhosis exclusively depicted on the HAP imaging on CT and MR imaging are pseudolesions or benign lesions particularly if they are small, wedge-shaped, and subcapsular in location.[141,142] Nevertheless, a high index of suspicion must be maintained in any cirrhotic patient with any focal hepatic lesion.

SUMMARY AND RECOMMENDATIONS

Ultimately the following 3 questions need to be answered in patients with incidental hepatic masses: (1) does the hepatic incidentaloma put the patient at risk for an adverse outcome? (2) can primary or metastatic malignancy be accurately and confidently differentiated from a benign incidentaloma? and (3) if a lesion is benign, might it still require surgical intervention, such as resecting a HA to prevent rupture?

The American College of Radiology has created a series of guidelines for the management of incidentally discovered hepatic masses discovered on cross-sectional imaging.[143] These guidelines are depicted in **Fig. 36** and are discussed here.

Managing incidental liver lesions depends on the probable importance of the mass. Importance is assessed based on the appearance of the mass and the level of risk that each patient has for developing significant liver masses, realizing that important liver masses are not limited to malignancies.

Patient risk for important hepatic masses is stratified as follows:

1. Low-risk individuals: Young patients ($\leq$40 years old), with no malignancy, hepatic dysfunction, hepatic malignant risk factors, or symptoms related to the liver
2. Average risk individuals: Patients older than 40 years, with no known malignancy, hepatic dysfunction, hepatic malignant risk factors, or symptoms related to the liver
3. High-risk individuals: Patients with a known primary malignancy with a propensity to metastasize to the liver, cirrhosis, and/or other hepatic risk factor. Hepatic risk factors include cirrhosis, hepatitis, chronic active hepatitis, sclerosing cholangitis, hemosiderosis, hepatic dysfunction, and long-term anabolic steroid or oral contraceptive use.

Using these guidelines, the vast majority of incidental lesions can be correctly characterized.

REFERENCES

1. Feinstein EG, Marr BP, Winston CB, et al. Hepatic abnormalities identified on abdominal computed tomography at diagnosis of uveal melanoma. Arch Ophthalmol 2010;128:319–23.
2. Tsung A, Geller DA. Workup of the incidental liver lesion. Adv Surg 2005;39:331–41.
3. Ather MH, Memon W, Rees J. Clinical impact of incidental diagnosis on non-contrast-enhanced helical CT for acute ureteral colic. Semin Ultrasound CT MR 2005;26:20–3.
4. Green DE, Woodward PJ. The management of indeterminate incidental findings detected at abdominal CT. Semin Ultrasound CT MR 2005;26:2–13.
5. Khan KY, Xiong T, McCafferty I, et al. Frequency and impact of extracolonic findings detected at computed tomographic colonography in a symptomatic population. Br J Surg 2007;94:355–61.
6. Sosna J, Kruskal JB, Bar-Ziv J, et al. Extracolonic findings at CT colonography. Abdom Imaging 2005;30:709–13.
7. Flicker MS, Tsoukas AT, Hazra A, et al. Economic impact of extracolonic findings at computed tomographic colonography. J Comput Assist Tomogr 2008;32:497–503.
8. Gluecker TM, Johnson CD, Wilson LA, et al. Extracolonic findings at CT colonography: evaluation of prevalence and cost in a screening population. Gastroenterology 2003;124:911–6.
9. Pilch-Kowalczyk J, Konopka M, Bibinska J, et al. Extracolonic findings at CT colonography—additional advantages of the method. Med Sci Monit 2004;10:22–5.

10. Hara AK, Johnson CD, MacCarty RL, et al. Incidental findings at CT colonography. Radiology 2000;215:353–7.

11. Hara AK. Extracolonic findings at CT colonography. Semin Ultrasound CT MR 2005;26:24–7.

12. Yee J, Kumar NN, Godara S, et al. Extracolonic abnormalities discovered incidentally at CT colonography in a male population. Radiology 2005; 236:519–26.

13. Xiong T, Richardson M, Woodroffe R, et al. Incidental lesions found on CT colonography: their nature and frequency. Br J Radiol 2005;78:22–9.

14. Spreng A, Netzer P, Mattich J, et al. Importance of extracolonic findings at IV contrast medium-enhanced CT colonography versus those at non-enhanced CT colonography. Eur Radiol 2005;15: 2088–95.

15. Hellström M, Svensson MH, Lasson A. Extracolonic and incidental findings on CT colonography (virtual colonoscopy). AJR Am J Roentgenol 2004;182: 631–8.

16. Salman R, Whiteley WN, Warlow C. Screening using whole-body magnetic resonance imaging scanning: who wants an incidentaloma? J Med Screen 2007;14:2–4.

17. Gil BN, Ran K, Tamar G, et al. Prevalence of significant noncardiac findings on coronary multidetector computed tomography angiography in asymptomatic patients. J Comput Assist Tomogr 2007;31:1–4.

18. Pickhard PJ, Taylor AJ. Extracolonic findings identified in asymptomatic adults at screening colonoscopy. AJR Am J Roentgenol 2006;186:718–28.

19. Seeff LB, Everson GT, Morgan TR, et al. Complication rate of percutaneous liver biopsies among persons with advanced chronic liver disease in the HALT-C trial. Clin Gastroenterol Hepatol 2010; 8:877–83.

20. Ros PR, Erturk SM. Benign tumors of the liver. In: Gore RM, Levine MS, editors. Textbook of gastrointestinal radiology. Philadelphia: Saunders; 2008. p. 1591–622.

21. Snover DC. Non-neoplastic liver disease. In: Mills EC, Carter D, Greeson JK, editors. Sternberg's diagnostic surgical pathology. 5th edition. Philadelphia: Lippincott Williams & Wilkins; 2009. p. 1167–91.

22. Washington K, Harris E. Masses of the liver. In: Mills EC, Carter D, Greeson JK, editors. Sternberg's diagnostic surgical pathology. 5th edition. Philadelphia: Lippincott Williams & Wilkins; 2009. p. 1192–2023.

23. Carrim ZI, Murchison JT. The prevalence of simple renal and hepatic cysts detected by spiral computed tomography. Clin Radiol 2003;58:626–9.

24. Oto A, Tamm EP, Zklaruk J. Multidetector row CT of the liver. Radiol Clin North Am 2005;43:827–48.

25. Rumack CM, Wilson SR, Charboneau W. The liver. In: Diagnostic ultrasound. 3rd edition. Philadelphia: Mosby; 2005. p. 678–801.

26. Braga L, Armao D, Semelka RC. Liver. In: Semelka RC, editor. Abdominal-pelvic MRI. 3rd edition. Hoboken (NJ): John Wiley; 2010. p. 347–446.

27. Mortele K, Peters HE. Multimodality imaging of common and uncommon cystic focal liver lesions. Semin Ultrasound CT MR 2009;30:368–86.

28. Cavallari A. Bile duct hamartomas: diagnostic problems and treatment. Hepatogastroenterology 1997;44:994–7.

29. Anderson SW, Kruskal JB, Kane RA. Benign hepatic tumors and iatrogenic pseudotumors. Radiographics 2009;29:211–29.

30. Brancatelli G, Federle MP, Vilgrain V, et al. Fibropolycystic liver disease: CT and MR imaging findings. Radiographics 2005;25:659–70.

31. Lev-Toaff AS, Bach AM, Wechsler RJ, et al. The radiologic and pathologic spectrum of biliary hamartomas. AJR Am J Roentgenol 1995;165: 309–13.

32. Cheung YC, Tan CF, Wan YL, et al. MRI of multiple biliary hamartomas. Br J Radiol 1997;70:527–9.

33. Mortele B, Mortele K, Seynaeve P, et al. Hepatic bile duct hamartomas (von Meyenburg complexes): MR and MR cholangiography findings. J Comput Assist Tomogr 2002;26:438–43.

34. Slone HW, Bennett WF, Bova JG. MR findings of multiple biliary hamartomas. AJR Am J Roentgenol 1993;161:581–3.

35. Choi BI, Lee JM. Neoplasms of the gallbladder and biliary tract. In: Gore RM, Levine MS, editors. Textbook of gastrointestinal radiology. 3rd edition. Philadelphia: Saunders; 2008. p. 1467–88.

36. Choi HK, Lee JK, Lee KH, et al. Differential diagnosis for intrahepatic biliary cystadenoma and hepatic simple cyst: significance of cystic fluid analysis and radiologic findings. J Clin Gastroenterol 2010;44:289–93.

37. Mortelé KJ, Ros PR. Cystic focal liver lesions in the adult: differential CT and MR imaging features. Radiographics 2001;21:895–910.

38. Tiniakos DG, Vos MB, Brunt EM. Nonalcoholic fatty liver disease: pathology and pathogenesis. Annu Rev Pathol 2010;5:145–71.

39. Gore RM. Diffuse liver disease. In: Gore RM, Levine MS, editors. Textbook of gastrointestinal radiology. 3rd edition. Philadelphia: Saunders; 2008. p. 1685–730.

40. Hamer OW, Aguirre DA, Casola G, et al. Fatty liver: imaging patterns and pitfalls. Radiographics 2006; 26:1637–53.

41. Tamai H, Shingaki N, Oka M, et al. Multifocal nodular fatty infiltration of the liver mimicking metastatic liver tumors. J Ultrasound Med 2006; 25:403–6.

42. Browning JD. New imaging techniques for non-alcoholic steatohepatitis. Clin Liver Dis 2009;13:607–19.

43. Desser TS. Understanding transient hepatic attenuation differences. Semin Ultrasound CT MR 2009;30:408–17.

44. Goshima S, Kanematsu M, Watanabe H, et al. Hepatic hemangioma and metastasis: differentiation with gadoxetate disodium-enhanced 3-T MRI. AJR Am J Roentgenol 2010;195:941–6.

45. Jang H-J, Kim TK, Lim HK. Hepatic hemangioma: atypical appearances on CT, MR imaging, and sonography. AJR Am J Roentgenol 2003;180:135–41.

46. Ma X, Holalkere NS, Kambadakone RA, et al. Imaging-based quantification of hepatic fat: methods and clinical applications. Radiographics 2009;29:1253–77.

47. Miyake H, Suzuki K, Ueda S, et al. Localized fat collection adjacent to the intrahepatic portion of the inferior vena cava: a normal variant on CT. AJR Am J Roentgenol 1992;158:423–5.

48. Perry JN, Williams MP, Dubbins PA, et al. Lipomata of the inferior vena cava: a normal variant? Clin Radiol 1994;49:341–2.

49. Han BK, Im JG, Jung JW, et al. Pericaval fat collection that mimics thrombosis of the inferior vena cava: demonstration with use of multi-directional reformation CT. Radiology 1997;203:105–8.

50. Hines J, Katz DS, Goffner L, et al. Fat collection related to the intrahepatic inferior vena cava on CT. AJR Am J Roentgenol 1999;172:409–11.

51. Baba Y, Hokotate H, Inoue H, et al. Pericaval fat mimicking intracaval deposits on unenhanced and contrast-enhanced helical CT in patients with cirrhosis. J Comput Assist Tomogr 2001;25:851–5.

52. Bioulac-Sage P, Laumonier H, Laurent C, et al. Benign and malignant vascular tumors of the liver in adults. Semin Liver Dis 2008;28:302–14.

53. Kamaya A, Maturen KE, Tye GA, et al. Hypervascular liver lesions. Semin Ultrasound CT MR 2009;30:387–407.

54. Arbiser JL, Bonner MY, Berrios RL. Hemangiomas, angiosarcomas, and vascular malformations represent the signaling abnormalities of pathogenic angiogenesis. Curr Mol Med 2009;9:929–34.

55. Dietrich CF, Mertens JC, Braden B, et al. Contrast-enhanced ultrasound of histologically proven liver hemangiomas. J Hepatol 2007;45:1139–45.

56. Kim KW, Kim AY, Kim TK, et al. Hepatic hemangiomas with arterioportal shunt: sonographic appearances with CT and MRI correlation. AJR Am J Roentgenol 2006;187:W406–14.

57. Kobayashi S, Maruyama H, Okugawa H, et al. Contrast-enhanced US with levovist for the diagnosis of hepatic hemangioma: time-related changes of enhancement appearance and the hemodynamic background. Hepatogastroenterology 2008;55:1222–8.

58. Yamashita Y, Ogata I, Urata J, et al. Cavernous hemangioma of the liver: pathologic correlation with dynamic CT findings. Radiology 1997;203:121–5.

59. Silva AC, Evans JM, McCullough AE, et al. MR imaging of hypervascular liver masses: a review of current techniques. Radiographics 2009;29:385–402.

60. Nguyen BN, Flejou JF, Terris B, et al. Focal nodular hyperplasia of the liver: a comprehensive pathologic study of 305 lesions and recognition of new histologic forms. Am J Surg Pathol 1999;23:1441–54.

61. Vilgrain V. Focal nodular hyperplasia. Eur J Radiol 2006;58:236–45.

62. Cherqui D, Rahmouni A, Charlotte F, et al. Management of focal nodular hyperplasia and hepatocellular adenoma in young women: a series of 41 patients with clinical, radiological, and pathological correlations. J Hepatol 1995;22:1674–81.

63. Kim MJ, Lim HK, Kim SH, et al. Evaluation of hepatic focal nodular hyperplasia with contrast-enhanced gray scale harmonic sonography: initial experience. J Ultrasound Med 2004;23:297–305.

64. van den Esschert JW, van Gulik TM, Phoa SS. Imaging modalities for focal nodular hyperplasia and hepatocellular adenoma. Dig Surg 2010;27:46–55.

65. Hussain SM, Terkivatan T, Zondervan PE, et al. Focal nodular hyperplasia: findings at state-of-the-art MR imaging, US, CT, and pathologic analysis. Radiographics 2004;24:3–17.

66. Kehagias D, Moulopoulos L, Antoniou A, et al. Focal nodular hyperplasia: imaging findings. Eur Radiol 2001;11:202–12.

67. Brancatelli G, Federle MP, Grazioli L, et al. Focal nodular hyperplasia: CT findings with emphasis on multiphasic helical CT in 78 patients. Radiology 2001;219:61–8.

68. Lin MC, Tsay PK, Ko SF, et al. Triphasic dynamic CT findings of 63 hepatic focal nodular hyperplasia in 46 patients: correlation with size and pathological findings. Abdom Imaging 2008;33:301–7.

69. Shirkhoda A, Farah MC, Bernacki E, et al. Hepatic focal nodular hyperplasia: CT and sonographic spectrum. Abdom Imaging 1994;19:34–8.

70. Caseiro-Alves F, Zins M, Mahfouz AE, et al. Calcification in focal nodular hyperplasia: a new problem for differentiation from fibrolamellar hepatocellular carcinoma. Radiology 1996;198:889–92.

71. Choi CS, Freeny PC. Triphasic helical CT of hepatic focal nodular hyperplasia: incidence of atypical findings. AJR Am J Roentgenol 1998;170:391–5.

72. Carlson SK, Johnson CD, Bender CE, et al. Of focal nodular hyperplasia of the liver. AJR Am J Roentgenol 2000;174:705–12.

73. Mortele KJ, Praet M, Van Vlierberghe H, et al. CT and MR imaging findings in focal nodular hyperplasia of the liver: radiologic-pathologic correlation. AJR Am J Roentgenol 2000;175:687–92.

74. Grazioli L, Morana G, Kirchin MA, et al. Accurate differentiation of focal nodular hyperplasia from hepatic adenoma at gadobenate dimeglumine-enhanced MR imaging: prospective study. Radiology 2005;236:166–77.

75. Ba-Ssalamah A, Schima W, Schmook MT, et al. Atypical focal nodular hyperplasia of the liver: imaging features of nonspecific and liver-specific MR contrast agents. AJR Am J Roentgenol 2002; 179:1447–56.

76. Kobayashi S, Matsui O, Gabata T, et al. Radiological and histopathological manifestations of hepatocellular nodular lesions concomitant with various congenital and acquired hepatic hemodynamic abnormalities. Jpn J Radiol 2009;27:53–68.

77. Golli M, Van Nhieu JT, Mathieu D, et al. Hepatocellular adenoma: color Doppler US and pathologic correlations. Radiology 1994;190:741–4.

78. Hussain SM, van den Bos IC, Dwarkasing RS, et al. Hepatocellular adenoma: findings at state-of-the-art magnetic resonance imaging, ultrasound, computed tomography and pathologic analysis. Eur Radiol 2006;16:1873–86.

79. Ichikawa T, Federle MP, Grazioli L, et al. Hepatocellular adenoma: multiphasic CT and histopathologic findings in 25 patients. Radiology 2000;214:861–8.

80. Arrive L, Flejou JF, Vilgrain V, et al. Hepatic adenoma: MR findings in 51 pathologically proved lesions. Radiology 1994;193:507–12.

81. Brancatelli G, Federle MP, Vullierme MP, et al. CT and MR imaging evaluation of hepatic adenoma. J Comput Assist Tomogr 2006;30:745–50.

82. Al-Mukhaizeem KA, Rosenberg A, Sherker AH. Nodular regenerative hyperplasia of the liver: an under-recognized cause of portal hypertension in hematological disorders. Am J Hematol 2004;75: 225–330.

83. Dachman AH, Ros PR, Goodman ZD, et al. Nodular regenerative hyperplasia of the liver: clinical and radiologic observations. AJR Am J Roentgenol 1987;148:717–22.

84. Siegelman ES, Outwater EK, Furth EE, et al. MR imaging of hepatic nodular regenerative hyperplasia. J Magn Reson Imaging 1995;5:730–2.

85. Ros PR, Taylor HM. Malignant tumors of the liver. In: Gore RM, Levine MS, editors. Textbook of gastrointestinal radiology. Philadelphia: WB Saunders; 2000. p. 1523–68.

86. Shariff MI, Cox IJ, Gomaa AI, et al. Hepatocellular carcinoma: current trends in worldwide epidemiology, risk factors, diagnosis and therapeutics. Expert Rev Gastroenterol Hepatol 2009; 3:353–67.

87. Schütte K, Bornschein J, Malfertheiner P. Hepatocellular carcinoma—epidemiological trends and risk factors. Dig Dis 2009;27:80–92.

88. Altekruse SF, McGlynn KA, Reichman ME. Hepatocellular carcinoma incidence, mortality, and survival trends in the United States from 1975 to 2005. J Clin Oncol 2009;20(27):1485–91.

89. Ahmed F, Perz JF, Kwong S, et al. National trends and disparities in the incidence of hepatocellular carcinoma, 1998–2003. Prev Chronic Dis 2008;5: 74–82.

90. Liu GJ, Wang W, Xie XY, et al. Real-time contrast-enhanced ultrasound imaging of focal liver lesions in fatty liver. Clin Imaging 2010;34:v211–21.

91. Lee MW, Kim YJ, Park HS, et al. Targeted sonography for small hepatocellular carcinoma discovered by CT or MRI: factors affecting sonographic detection. AJR Am J Roentgenol 2010;194:W396–400.

92. Colli A, Fraquelli M, Casazza G, et al. Accuracy of ultrasonography, spiral CT, magnetic resonance, and alpha-fetoprotein in diagnosing hepatocellular carcinoma: a systematic review. Am J Gastroenterol 2006;101:513–23.

93. Baron RL, Brancatelli G. Computed tomographic imaging of hepatocellular carcinoma. Gastroenterology 2004;127(Suppl 1):S133–43.

94. Laghi A, Iannaccone R, Rossi P, et al. Hepatocellular carcinoma: detection with triple-phase multidetector row helical CT in patients with chronic hepatitis. Radiology 2003;226:543–9.

95. Mitsuzaki K, Yamashita Y, Ogata I, et al. Multiple-phase helical CT of the liver for detecting small hepatomas in patients with liver cirrhosis: contrast-injection protocol and optimal timing. AJR Am J Roentgenol 1996;167:753–7.

96. Monzawa S, Ichikawa T, Nakajima H, et al. Dynamic CT for detecting small hepatocellular carcinoma: usefulness of delayed phase imaging. AJR Am J Roentgenol 2007;188:147–53.

97. Willatt JM, Hussain HK, Adusumilli S, et al. MR imaging of hepatocellular carcinoma in the cirrhotic liver: challenges and controversies. Radiology 2008;247:311–30.

98. Cabibbo G, Craxì A. Epidemiology, risk factors and surveillance of hepatocellular carcinoma. Eur Rev Med Pharmacol Sci 2010;14:352–5.

99. Wong LK, Link DP, Frey CF, et al. Fibrolamellar hepatocarcinoma: radiology, management, and pathology. AJR Am J Roentgenol 1982;139:172–5.

100. Smith MT, Blatt ER, Jedlicka P, et al. Best cases from the AFIP: fibrolamellar hepatocellular carcinoma. Radiographics 2008;28:609–13.

101. McLarney JK, Rucker PT, Bender GN, et al. Fibrolamellar carcinoma of the liver: radiologic-pathologic correlation. Radiographics 1999;19:453–71.

102. Terzis I, Haritanti A, Economou I. Fibrolamellar hepatocellular carcinoma: a case report with

distinct radiological features. J Gastrointest Cancer 2010;41:2–5.

103. Bedi DG, Kumar R, Morettin LB, et al. Fibrolamellar carcinoma of the liver: CT, ultrasound and angiography. Eur J Radiol 1988;8:109–12.

104. Abrams HL, Giordano TJ, Brodeur FJ, et al. Metastases in carcinoma: analysis of 1000 autopsied cases. Cancer 1950;3:74–85.

105. Primrose JN. Surgery for colorectal liver metastases. Br J Cancer 2010;102:1313–8.

106. Namasivayam S, Martin DR, Saini S. Imaging of liver metastases: MRI. Cancer Imaging 2007;7:2–9.

107. Ahn JH, Yu JS, Hwang SH, et al. Nontumorous arterioportal shunts in the liver: CT and MRI findings considering mechanisms and fate. Eur Radiol 2010;20:385–94.

108. Colegrande S, Centi N, Galdiero R, et al. Transient hepatic intensity differences: part 1. Those associated with focal lesions. AJR Am J Roentgenol 2007; 188:154–9.

109. Colegrande S, Centi N, Galdiero R, et al. Transient hepatic intensity differences: part 2. Those not associated with focal lesions. AJR Am J Roentgenol 2007;188:160–6.

110. Eberhardt SC, Choi PH, Bach AM, et al. Utility of sonography for small hepatic lesions found on computed tomography in patients with cancer. J Ultrasound Med 2003;22:335–43.

111. Kim HJ, Kim AY, Kim TK, et al. Transient hepatic attenuation differences in focal hepatic lesions: dynamic CT features. AJR Am J Roentgenol 2005;184:83–90.

112. Colegrande S, Centi N, La Villa G, et al. Transient hepatic attenuation differences. AJR Am J Roentgenol 2004;183:459–64.

113. Lee KH, Han JK, Jeong JY, et al. Hepatic attenuation differences associated with obstruction of the portal or hepatic veins in patients with hepatic abscesses. AJR Am J Roentgenol 2005;185:1015–23.

114. Choi SH, Lee JM, Lee KH, et al. Relationship between various patterns of transient hepatic attenuation on CT and portal vein thrombosis related to acute cholecystitis. AJR Am J Roentgenol 2004;183:437–42.

115. Yoshimoto K, Honda H, Kuriowa T, et al. Unusual hemodynamics and pseudolesions of the noncirrhotic liver at CT. Radiographics 2001;881–96.

116. Quiroag S, Sebastia C, Pallisa E, et al. Improved diagnosis of hepatic perfusion disorders: value of hepatic arterial phase imaging during helical CT. Radiographics 2001;21:65–81.

117. Colagrande S, Centi N, Pradella S, et al. Transient hepatic attenuation differences and focal liver lesions: sump effect due to primary arterial hyperperfusion. J Comput Assist Tomogr 2009;33:259–65.

118. Yamasaki M, Furukawa A, Murata K, et al. Transient hepatic attenuation difference (THAD) in patients without neoplasm: frequency, shape, distribution, and causes. Radiat Med 1999;17(2):91–6.

119. Ito K, Awaya H, Mitchell DG, et al. Gallbladder disease: appearance of associated transient increased attenuation in the liver at biphasic, contrast-enhanced dynamic CT. Radiology 1997; 204:723–8.

120. Chen WP, Chen JH, Hwang JI, et al. Spectrum of transient hepatic attenuation differences in biphasic helical CT. AJR Am J Roentgenol 1999;172:419–24.

121. Catalano O, Sandomenico F, Nunziata A, et al. Transient hepatic echogenicity difference on contrast-enhanced ultrasonography: sonographic sign and pitfall. J Ultrasound Med 2007;26:337–45.

122. Hwang SH, Yu JS, Chung J, et al. Transient hepatic attenuation difference (THAD) following transcatheter arterial chemoembolization for hepatic malignancy: changes on serial CT examinations. Eur Radiol 2008;18(1):596–603.

123. Yamashita K, Jin MJ, Hirose Y, et al. CT finding of transient focal increased attenuation of the liver adjacent to the gallbladder in acute cholecystitis. AJR Am J Roentgenol 1995;164:343–6.

124. Tian JL, Zhang JS. Hepatic perfusion disorders: etiopathogenesis and related diseases. World J Gastroenterol 2006;12:3265–70.

125. Gabata T, Kadoya M, Matsui O, et al. Dynamic CT of hepatic abscesses: significance of transient segmental enhancement. AJR Am J Roentgenol 2001;176:675–9.

126. Pradella S, Centi N, La Villa G, et al. Transient hepatic attenuation difference (THAD) in biliary duct disease. Abdom Imaging 2009;34:626–33.

127. Soyer P, Devine N, Somveille E, et al. Hepatic pseudolesion around the falciform ligament: prevalence on CT examination. Abdom Imaging 1996;21:324–8.

128. Yoshimitsu K, Honda H, Kuroiwa T, et al. Pseudolesions of the liver possibly caused by focal rib compression: analysis based on hemodynamic change. AJR Am J Roentgenol 1999;172:645–9.

129. Bertolotto M, Martinoli C, Migaleddu V, et al. Color Doppler sonography of intrahepatic vascular shunts. J Clin Ultrasound 2008;36:527–38.

130. Khalid SK, Garcia-Tsao G. Hepatic vascular malformations in hereditary hemorrhagic telangiectasia. Semin Liver Dis 2008;28:247–58.

131. Danet IM, Semelka RC, Leonardou P, et al. Spectrum of MRI appearances of untreated metastases of the liver. AJR Am J Roentgenol 2003;181:809–17.

132. Sica GT, Ji H, Ros PR. CT and MR imaging of hepatic metastases. AJR Am J Roentgenol 2000; 174:691–8.

133. Holalkere N-J, Sahani DV, Blake MA, et al. Characterization of small liver lesions: added role of MR after MDCT. J Comput Assist Tomogr 2006;30:591–6.

134. Lim GH, Koh DC, Cheong WK, et al. Natural history of small, "indeterminate" hepatic lesions in patients

with colorectal cancer. Dis Colon Rectum 2009;52: 1487–91.

135. Patterson SA, Khalil HI, Panicek DM. MRI evaluation of small hepatic lesions in women with breast cancer. AJR Am J Roentgenol 2006;187:307–12.

136. Jones EC, Chezmar JL, Nelson RC, et al. The frequency and significance of small (less than or equal to 15 mm) hepatic lesions detected by CT. AJR Am J Roentgenol 1992;158:535–9.

137. Schwartz LH, Gandras EJ, Colangelo S, et al. Prevalence and importance of small hepatic lesions found at CT in patients with cancer. Radiology 1999;210:71–4.

138. Jang HJ, Lim HK, Lee WJ, et al. Small hypoattenuating lesions in the liver on single-phase helical CT in preoperative patients with gastric and colorectal cancer: prevalence, significance, and differentiating features. J Comput Assist Tomogr 2002;26: 718–24.

139. Khalil HI, Patterson SA, Panicek DM. Hepatic lesions deemed too small to characterize at CT: prevalence and importance in women with breast cancer. Radiology 2005;235:872–8.

140. Krakora GA, Coakley FV, Williams G, et al. Small hypoattenuating hepatic lesions at contrast-enhanced CT: prognostic importance in patients with breast cancer. Radiology 2004;233:667–73.

141. Hwang SH, Yu JS, Kim KW, et al. Small hypervascular enhancing lesions on arterial phase images of multiphase dynamic computed tomography in cirrhotic liver: fate and implications. J Comput Assist Tomogr 2008;32:39–45.

142. Holland AE, Hecht EM, Hahn WY, et al. Importance of small ($\leq$20-mm) enhancing lesions seen only during the hepatic arterial phase at MR imaging of the cirrhotic liver: evaluation and comparison with whole explanted liver. Radiology 2005;237: 938–44.

143. Berland LL, Silverman SG, Gore RM, et al. Managing incidental findings on abdominal CT: white paper of the ACR Incidental Finding Committee. J Am Coll Radiol 2010;7:754–73.

Splenic Incidentalomas

Sameer Ahmed[a], Karen M. Horton, MD[b],*,
Elliot K. Fishman, MD[c]

KEYWORDS

• Spleen • Incidentalomas • Computed tomography

The spleen is often referred to as the forgotten organ. This claim may be because the spleen is not necessary for survival, although it certainly plays an important role in immunity. Its exact functions are still a mystery. Compared with other intraabdominal organs such as the liver and pancreas, there is a significant paucity of scientific investigation involving the spleen. This situation is especially true in the radiology literature, in which little has been published regarding the detection and characterization of splenic disease conditions.

Splenic lesions are common in a busy radiology practice. Technical advancements in computed tomography (CT) now allow unprecedented temporal and spatial resolution; unexpected splenic lesions are commonly detected on CT examinations of the abdomen and chest and often pose a diagnostic challenge to both the radiologist and clinician. This article discusses incidental splenic lesions detected on CT and explores potential management strategies.

INCIDENTAL SPLENIC LESIONS

Data on the prevalence of splenic incidentalomas are limited. Two studies conducted at level I trauma centers have reported the prevalence of incidental splenic lesions detected on CT.

In a study of 3113 patients at a level I trauma center, Ekeh and colleagues[1] reported on the prevalence of various incidentally detected lesions on abdominal CT. Scanning was performed on a GE Hi-Speed 4-Slice scanner with intravenous (IV) contrast. The prevalence of splenic granuloma and accessory spleen was 1.38% and 0.1%, respectively. The detection rates of splenic cyst and splenic hemangioma were each less than 0.08%. All incidentally detected splenic lesions in this study were benign.[1] Another recent study at a level I trauma center reported only 10 cases of incidental splenic findings on high-definition spiral CT from a total of 991 patients.[2] This study included cases of splenic cyst (4), splenomegaly (4), splenic hemangioma (one), and splenic abscess (one), with a total prevalence of only 1.0%. All reported lesions were considered clinically benign.

These 2 studies are relevant because lesions detected in the spleen were truly incidental, because these were patients being scanned for trauma. In clinical practice, when splenic lesions are detected, it is sometimes difficult to be sure that they are incidental findings, especially in patients being scanned for vague abdominal symptoms.

CT IMAGING OF THE SPLEEN

Before discussing individual splenic lesions, it is important to briefly discuss the normal appearance of the spleen on CT as well as technical issues related to CT imaging of the spleen.

The spleen is an intraperitoneal organ with a smooth serosal surface. Splenic clefts are common as a result of incomplete fusion of the embryonic splenic buds, and should not be

[a] Johns Hopkins School of Medicine, 1620 McElderry Street, Baltimore, MD 21205, USA
[b] Russell H. Morgan Department of Radiology and Radiological Science, Johns Hopkins Medical Institutions, JHOC 3253, 601 North Caroline Street, Baltimore, MD 21287, USA
[c] Russell H. Morgan Department of Radiology and Radiological Science, Johns Hopkins Medical Institutions, JHOC 3254, 601 North Caroline Street, Baltimore, MD 21287-0801, USA
* Corresponding author.
E-mail address: kmhorton@jhmi.edu

Radiol Clin N Am 49 (2011) 323–347
doi:10.1016/j.rcl.2010.11.001

interpreted as laceration or previous infarcts (Fig. 1).[3] Similarly, spenules (unfused splenic buds) are common and have been reported to occur in 10% of the population (Fig. 2).[4] These accessory spleens should not be mistaken for adenopathy, implants, or masses in adjacent organs such as the pancreas or left adrenal gland.[5]

In addition, because of the presence of white pulp and red pulp, there are variable circulatory routes through the spleen. This situation results in heterogeneous perfusion of the spleen after IV contrast administration.[6] This pattern often seems serpentine or chordlike (Fig. 3). It is more common early after rapid contrast administration and is exaggerated in patients with portal hypertension, splenic vein occlusion, or heart failure. This early enhancement pattern can obscure an underlying splenic mass or laceration. Alternatively, the heterogeneous appearance can simulate the presence of focal splenic masses.

The best time to image the spleen after IV contrast administration has not been well established. However, if a CT is being performed to characterize a known or suspected splenic lesion, there are some guidelines. It is probably reasonable to obtain a noncontrast scan to better define the presence of calcifications or hemorrhage and to obtain a baseline density of the lesion. After IV contrast administration (3–5 mL/s), an arterial scan at 30 s is useful to better define vascularity and enhancement as well as to visualize the splenic artery. The parenchyma of the spleen may not be well imaged at this time. A later phase scan at 60 to 70 s is helpful to show homogeneous parenchymal enhancement and to allow more accurate detection of small lesions. Delayed scans may be of value in select cases.

The role of three-dimensional imaging for evaluation and characterization of splenic lesions has not been well studied. However, the ability to visualize the spleen and splenic diseases in more than one plane has been useful in our clinical practice (Fig. 4).

CLINICAL CORRELATION

The CT appearances of a variety of splenic lesions overlap considerably. When a splenic lesion is detected on CT, it often cannot be characterized completely without basic clinical correlation. For example, is it truly an incidental lesion in an asymptomatic patient? Does the patient have pain that could be related to the spleen? Does the patient have a fever? Is the patient immunocompromised? Does the patient have an underlying malignancy? Does the patient have a history of trauma? Is there an isolated splenic lesion or multiple splenic lesions? Is there any other associated abdominal condition, such as liver lesions or adenopathy? This information is critical when evaluating splenic disease. The appearances of splenic lesions on CT are typically not pathognomonic and often cannot be characterized based on the CT appearance alone.

PATIENT SCENARIOS

This section presents a series of clinical scenarios involving splenic lesions detected on CT. Each scenario includes a discussion of the relevant

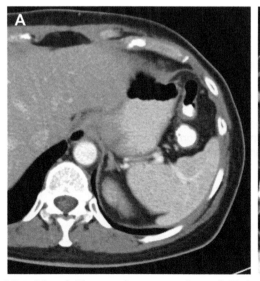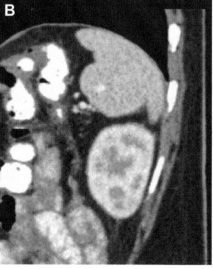

Fig. 1. (A) Axial and (B) coronal contrast-enhanced CT shows a splenic cleft along the posterior and inferior margin.

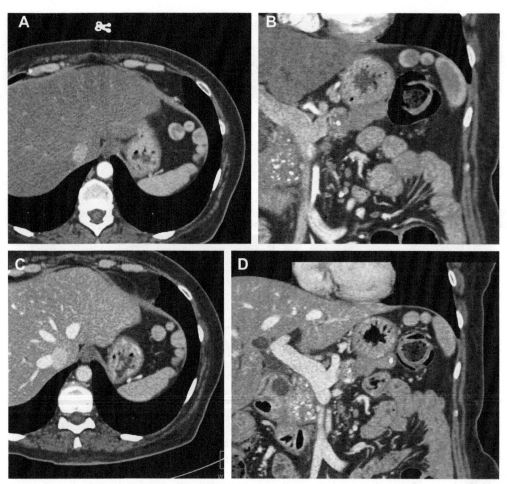

Fig. 2. 50-year-old woman with chronic pancreatitis. Contrast-enhanced CT in the arterial (*A, B*) and venous (*C, D*) phases show small spenules near the upper pole of the spleen. Notice how the splenules enhance similarly to the spleen.

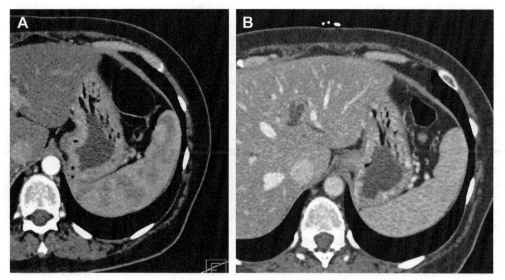

Fig. 3. Normal enhancement pattern of the spleen in the arterial (*A*) and venous (*B*) phases.

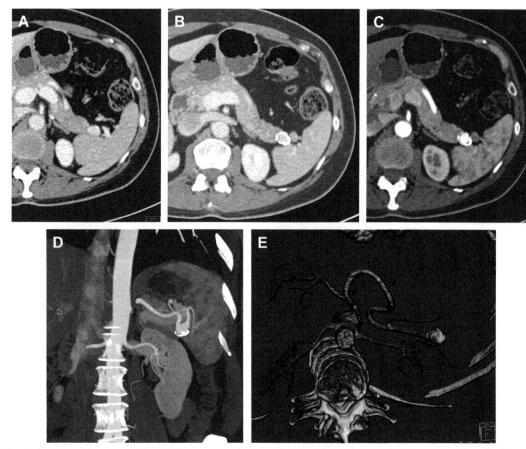

Fig. 4. 55-year-old woman referred from an outside hospital for islet cell tumor in the pancreatic tail, diagnosed on an outside CT. The outside CT was performed in the venous phase only (not shown). Repeat CT in the venous phase (*A, B*) shows a 2-cm enhancing lesion in the pancreatic tail with peripheral calcification. Arterial phase images in the (*C*) axial plane show the lesion to be vascular. (*D*) Coronal maximum intensity projection and (*E*) volume rendering show a splenic artery aneurysm.

differential diagnosis as well as management suggestions and teaching points.

Splenic Calcification

A 30-year-old woman underwent a noncontrast CT for right flank pain and suspected renal calculi. Multiple punctate calcifications were noted in the spleen (Fig. 5).

This CT appearance is classic for previous granulomatous disease involving the spleen. In most cases, multiple punctate splenic calcifications represent healed granulomatous disease, the most common of which in North America is histoplasmosis.[7] The organism is transmitted through inhalation of soil infected with bird or bat excrement. There may also be associated calcifications in the liver, abdominal lymph nodes, and/or mediastinal and hilar nodes.

In immunocompromised patients, *Pneumocystis carinii* has been reported, often in patients with

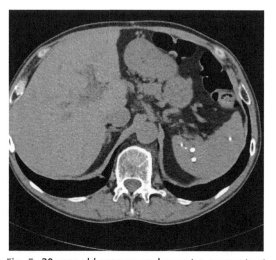

Fig. 5. 30-year-old woman underwent a noncontrast CT for right flank pain and suspected renal calculi. Multiple punctate calcifications were noted in the spleen compatible with previous granulomatous disease.

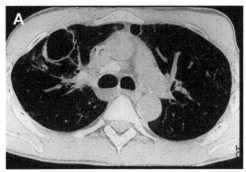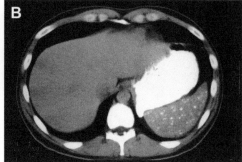

Fig. 6. Patient with AIDS and previous disseminated pneumocystis infection. (A) Chest CT shows pneumatoceles from previous PCP. (B) Noncontrast CT through the spleen shows characteristic calcifications.

Mycobacterium avium-intracellulare complex.[8] This infection can result in multiple small calcifications in the spleen and liver during both active and resolved infections and is often associated with splenomegaly[8] (Fig. 6).

Other causes of splenic calcification include sickle cell disease (Fig. 7), and healed infarcts (Fig. 8). Calcifications can occur in splenic cysts, hamartomas, hemangiomas, hydatid disease, or healed abscesses. Typically there is a clinical history to support these entities.

Teaching point

Multiple punctate calcifications in the spleen are a common finding on CT. They are usually associated with similar calcifications in the liver and lymph nodes, but not always. In most patients these calcifications represent healed granulomatous disease, most commonly histoplasmosis or tuberculosis. No further work-up is needed. This condition is typically reported as healed granulomatous disease. In immunocompromised patients, disseminated *Pneumocystis carinii* could have a similar appearance, but it is rarely seen.

Splenic Cyst

A 43-year-old woman with recurrent urinary tract infections and hematuria underwent a multiphase CT (Fig. 9). In this patient, there is an incidental sharply defined 3-cm low-density splenic lesion. No enhancement was noted after IV contrast. This appearance is characteristic of a benign cyst.

Relatively benign in nature, splenic cysts are usually an incidental finding on radiologic examination, surgery, or autopsy, but some larger cysts may present with abdominal pain and gastrointestinal symptoms.[9] In a study of splenic epidermoid cysts in children by Tsakayannis and colleagues,[10] only cysts larger than 8 cm in diameter presented with symptoms. Some rare complications include hemorrhage, rupture, or superimposed infection, resulting in symptoms.[9,11]

Splenic cysts are classified into 2 major subtypes: true cysts and false cysts (posttraumatic

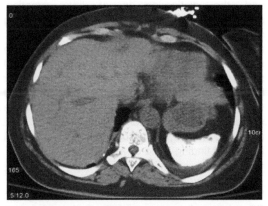

Fig. 7. Noncontrast CT in a patient with sickle cell disease shows a small densely calcified spleen.

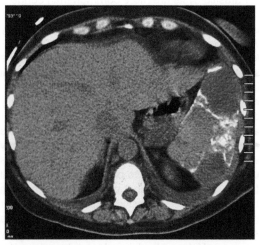

Fig. 8. Noncontrast CT through the upper abdomen shows segmental and geographic areas of calcification, compatible with healed infarcts.

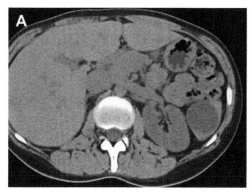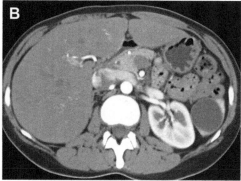

Fig. 9. 43-year-old woman with recurrent urinary tract infection and hematuria, who underwent a CT. There is a 3-cm cyst in the spleen. This cyst measured 15 HU on noncontrast examination (A). No enhancement was noted after IV contrast (B). This finding is compatible with a cyst. It is not always possible to distinguish a true cyst from a false cyst on CT.

pseudocysts). This differentiation is based on the presence or absence of an epithelial lining. True cysts, which constitute approximately 20% of all splenic cysts and show an epithelial lining, are further divided into nonparasitic cysts and parasitic subtypes. Nonparasitic, true cysts, primarily known as epidermoid cysts, are congenitally derived from peritoneal mesothelium[6,9] and represent only 2.5% of all splenic cysts.[10] On multidetector CT (MDCT), epidermoid cysts are well-defined, low-density, low-attenuating lesions that typically present as a unilocular mass with a thin or imperceptible wall.[9,12] Their attenuation is equal to that of water and no appreciable contrast enhancement is observed, except possibly in the internal trabeculae.[6,9] Approximately 86% of true cysts show Cyst-wall trabeculations or peripheral septations on MDCT.[13] Cyst-wall calcifications are observed on CT in 14% of true cysts.[13]

Parasitic cysts are more common than congenital epidermoid cysts, worldwide, but are extremely rare in the United States. Infection by *Tenia echinococcus*, usually *Echinococcus granulosus*, is the primary cause of parasitic cysts in the spleen. However, the major sites of echinococcal infection are the liver and lungs.[11] Splenic involvement in an echinococcal infection is usually caused by either systemic dissemination or a ruptured hepatic cyst.[9] Although parasitic cysts are the most prevalent true cysts worldwide, they are rarely found in Western countries.[10] It is unusual for these cysts to present as an incidental finding, especially without evidence of disease in the lungs or liver. Parasitic splenic cysts appear homogeneous on CT, with attenuation levels similar to that of epidermoid cysts and high density because of intracystic debris, hydatid sand, and/or inflammation.[14,15] Calcification in the wall of the cyst may become visible after death of the parasite. Cysts of parasitic origin should be suspected in patients from areas of endemic hydatid disease (Argentina, Greece, and Spain) with concurrent liver cysts and positive serologic findings.[9,12]

False cysts, also known as posttraumatic pseudocysts, lack an epithelial lining and are considered to represent the end stage of a previous intrasplenic hematoma. They account for up to 80% of all splenic cysts.[12] Patients may report a history of trauma to the left upper quadrant, but up to 30% of patients do not recall any association with such an event.[11,12] Previous infarction or infection of the spleen may also contribute to the incidence of false cysts.[11] These lesions appear nearly identical to true cysts on CT scans. However, only approximately 17% of false cysts show cyst-wall trabeculations or peripheral septations on MDCT.[13] Cyst-wall calcifications are more common in false cysts compared with true cysts, occurring in up to 50% of cases[13] (Fig. 10).

It is usually impossible to distinguish between true and false cysts on radiologic examination and the distinction is of little practical significance.[6,9] MDCT is useful in differentiating a cyst (true or false) from a malignant splenic neoplasm or abscess. The treatment approach to splenic cysts is dependent on lesion size and symptoms. Generally, symptomatic cysts or lesions larger than 5 cm in diameter are managed with spleen-preserving minimally invasive surgery.[11] Larger symptomatic cysts require splenectomy. Smaller, asymptomatic cysts are truly an incidental finding of no clinical significance.

Teaching point
Splenic cysts are common incidental findings on CT. It is usually not possible to distinguish a true from a false cyst and it is not clinically important

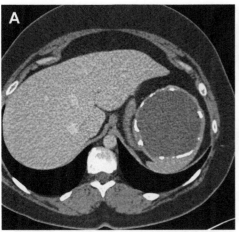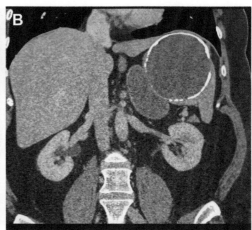

Fig. 10. 50-year-old woman with remote history of cervical cancer. CT was performed for evaluation of left upper quadrant pain. (A, B) CT reveals a 9-cm splenic cyst with dense peripheral calcification, compatible with a pseudo-cyst. Because of persistent pain and gastric compression, splenectomy was performed. Investigation revealed a pseudocyst related to a calcified hematoma. The patient denied history of trauma.

to try to do so. These cysts are reported as benign splenic cysts. Other splenic lesions can be cystic. For example, some metastases appear cystic, such as ovarian metastases, but as discussed later, isolated splenic metastases are uncommon, and these patients almost always have other sites of metastases. Splenic abscesses can appear cystic but may also have an enhancing rim or air within the lesion to help distinguish them from benign cysts (Fig. 11). The walls may be thickened or less well defined. Also it is unusual to detect an incidental splenic abscess, because these patients are typically very sick.

Splenic Hemangioma

A 61-year-old man undergoing abdominal CT for mildly increased results in liver function

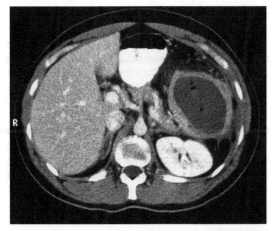

Fig. 11. Contrast-enhanced CT shows a thick-walled collection in the spleen with air, compatible with a splenic abscess.

tests. CT reveals a 3-cm enhancing lesion in the spleen (Fig. 12). This lesion was also present on a scan from 5 years previously. No other lesions were noted in the spleen or liver. Given the CT appearance and stability, this lesion is likely a hemangioma.

Splenic hemangioma is the most common benign primary neoplasm of the spleen, with prevalence at autopsy ranging from 0.3% to 14%.[16] This large variation is a result of a lack of distinction by some investigators between various benign vascular lesions. Congenital in origin, hemangiomas arise from sinusoidal epithelium and are composed of numerous vascular channels containing slow-flowing blood. Cavernous hemangioma is the predominant subtype and is typically detected in adults between 30 and 50 years of age.[17] Multiple lesions can be observed in cases of systemic angiomatosis (Klippel-Trenauney-Weber, Beckwith-Wiedemann, and Turner syndromes)[18] (Fig. 13). Hemangiomas are typically 1 to 2 cm in diameter, but can vary in size from a few millimeters to several centimeters.[19]

Splenic hemangiomas are slow growing and usually an incidental finding in patients undergoing radiologic and pathologic examinations.[9] Several studies have presented cases of incidental splenic hemangiomas on CT[20,21] but the prevalence is currently unknown. Patients may present with pain over the left upper quadrant and gastrointestinal disturbance (diarrhea, constipation, and/or dysphagia) in late adulthood. Anemia, thrombocytopenia, and coagulopathy are associated with lesions of increasing size. However, most are asymptomatic.[16,20]

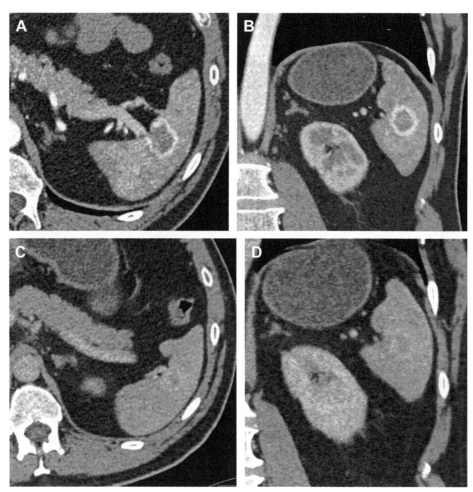

Fig. 12. 61-year-old man undergoing abdominal CT for mildly increased results in liver function tests. Arterial phase images in the axial (A) and coronal plane (B) show a 3-cm low-density lesion with peripheral enhancement. (C, D) Venous phase images show progressive enhancement. The lesion was also present 5 years previously (not shown). Given the CT appearance and stability, this lesion is likely a hemangioma.

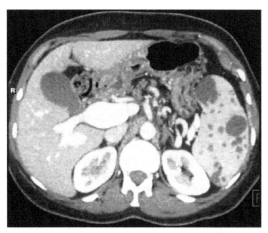

Fig. 13. Contrast-enhanced CT in a patient with Klippel-Trenauney-Weber syndrome shows multiple low-density splenic lesions compatible with multiple hemangiomata.

Although these lesions are relatively benign in nature, the most common complication is spontaneous rupture, which may evolve into a life-threatening condition. The prevalence of rupture was reported to occur in up to 25% of cases in a 56-patient series,[22] but this complication is less common with early detection on radiologic examination.

The appearance of hemangiomas on CT is variable. Hemangiomas present as a spectrum of solid to cystic lesions on MDCT. Without contrast, solid regions appear hypodense or isodense with the normal spleen.[17] Increased attenuation of the mass from periphery to center can be observed on administration of contrast material[9] (see Fig. 12). Low-density lesions show peripheral enhancement on MDCT.[23] In most cases, cavernous hemangiomas show a mixture of cystic and solid components, whereas only the solid regions exhibit contrast enhancement.[23] In the late phase of contrast, splenic hemangiomas rarely show the typical centripetal enhancement seen in similar hepatic lesions. Solid regions present with central punctate calcifications, whereas curvilinear calcifications are seen in the periphery of cystic portions.[12] Appearance on CT also varies with size because larger lesions may show evidence of fibrosis, infarction, and pseudocystic degeneration resulting from necrosis.[23] Some lesions may be avascular and show slow filling of contrast media.[9] Other lesions may show hyper enhancement on early phase and be isointense on delayed imaging (**Fig. 14**).

Treatment of symptomatic splenic hemangioma most often consists of splenectomy.[24]

Teaching point
An incidentally detected vascular splenic lesion usually represents a hemangioma. As discussed earlier, the CT enhancement pattern can be similar to the characteristic enhancement pattern of hepatic hemangiomata, but typically is not. In the absence of symptoms and without evidence of hemorrhage, no further imaging is needed. If the patient is symptomatic or there is CT evidence of hemorrhage and/or associated hepatic vascular

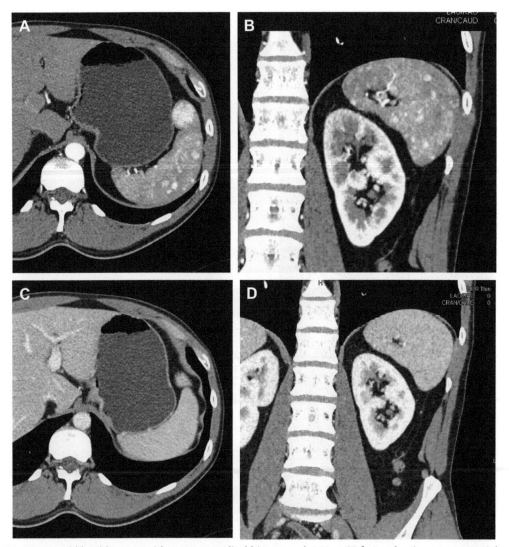

Fig. 14. 36-year-old healthy man with no past medical history underwent CT for evaluation as a potential renal donor. Arterial phase images in the (*A*) axial and (*B*) coronal plane show multiple small enhancing lesions throughout the spleen. The lesions are not visible on the venous phase images (*C*) and (*D*). The remainder of the CT of the abdomen and pelvis was normal. These lesions are presumed hemangiomata. The patient was a successful donor.

lesions, then further investigation is warranted. The lesions could represent vascular metastases within the liver and spleen or a primary angiosarcoma of the spleen with liver metastases. However, angiosarcoma of the spleen is rare.

Splenic Hamartoma

A 64-year-old patient undergoing CT for evaluation of elevated liver enzymes. CT reveals a 2-cm low-density lesion seen at the upper pole of the spleen (Fig. 15). This lesion is better appreciated on the early scan. The CT appearance is compatible with a hamartoma.

Splenic hamartoma is a rare, benign tumor, characterized by a well-circumscribed, solid, nodular appearance.[23] They are unencapsulated and may infiltrate into surrounding compressed splenic tissue, with focal or diffuse fibrosis.[25] Hamartomas are divided into 2 subtypes: white and red pulp lesions, based on architecture. White pulp lesions contain aberrant lymphoid tissue. The red pulp subtype is composed of an irregular complex of sinuses and structures that are analogous to the pulp cords of normal splenic tissue.[22] Most hamartomas are a mixture of the 2 subtypes. Their incidence on autopsy series ranges from 0.024% to 0.13% and is usually discovered as an incidental finding on radiologic examination, autopsy, or

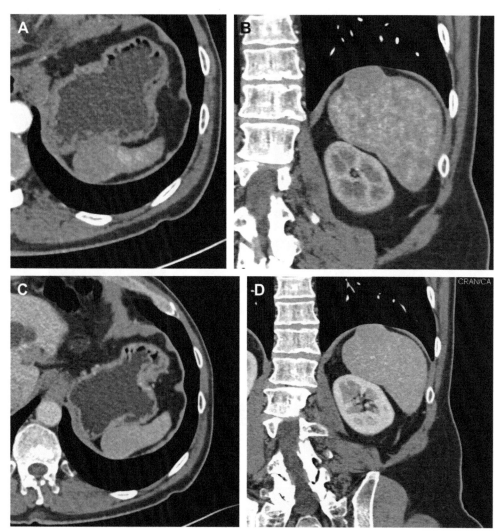

Fig. 15. 64-year-old patient undergoing CT for evaluation of elevated liver enzymes. Arterial phase images in the (*A*) axial and coronal (*B*) plane show the normal early enhancement pattern of the spleen. There is a 2-cm low-density lesion seen at the upper pole of the spleen. Venous phase images in the (*C*) axial and (*D*) coronal plane again show the lesion, but it is less apparent except for a contour defect. The CT appearance is compatible with a hamartoma.

exploratory laparotomy.[9,21] Hamartomas are associated with tuberous sclerosis and Wiskott-Aldrich-like syndrome, and some evidence suggests that they may be congenital in origin.[22] Rare associations with anemia and thrombocytopenia have also been shown in case studies, especially among younger patients, likely because of sequestration of hematopoietic cells.[26,27]

Most splenic hamartomas are discovered incidentally in asymptomatic patients, without any gender or age predilection. However, an estimated 15% of lesions present with abdominal discomfort, fever, malaise, splenomegaly, and/or portal hypertension.[26] Spontaneous splenic rupture has been reported in rare instances.[28] In a study by Lam and colleagues,[29] 3 of 6 splenic hamartomas showed association with neoplastic disorders.

On MDCT, hamartomas appear as an irregularity in the contour of the spleen. They are iso- or hypoattenuating on nonenhanced CT scans and can be difficult to detect. After administration of contrast media, prolonged enhancement is observed on CT, largely attributed to stagnant flow within the aberrant sinusoids of the red pulp.[9,30] This is a useful finding in differentiating hamartoma from malignant lesions of the spleen, especially nodular lymphoma.[30] When observed on CT, a hamartoma appears as a well-defined mass with smooth borders, and usually without infiltration of the surrounding parenchyma. However, in some cases, a nondescript contour abnormality may be the only finding on CT,[17] especially on delayed imaging. Complete or partial splenectomy is the most frequent course of treatment if the patient is symptomatic or in cases of rupture.[31]

Teaching point

Splenic hamartomas are rare. They should be considered when solid splenic lesions are noted in patients with tuberous sclerosis and Wiskott-Aldrich-like syndrome, given the increased incidence. They should also be considered in younger patients with thrombocytopenia. Malignant lesions, like lymphoma and metastasis, may have a similar appearance, but a clinical history is expected to support those diagnoses.

Splenic Lymphangioma

A 46-year-old woman underwent hysterectomy for fibroids. During the procedure, the surgeon noted splenomegaly and multiple splenic lesions. No biopsy was performed. Contrast-enhanced CT was performed and showed splenomegaly with multiple cystic lesions throughout the enlarged spleen (Fig. 16). No enhancement of the lesions
was noted. Hematologic work-up suggested that she had minimal residual splenic function. The patient now complained of mild pain. Splenectomy was performed and investigation revealed lymphangiomatosis.

Splenic lymphangioma is a rare, benign tumor composed of multiple vascular channels that are lined with a single layer of flattened endothelium and contain proteinaceous fluid (lymph).[9] They are considered congenital malformations with obstruction or agenesis of lymphatic tissue that leads to limited communication with the lymphatic system.[32] This lesion is classified by size and location of vascular channels into 3 subtypes: cystic, simple (capillary), and cavernous.[33] Their pathologic appearance ranges from single and multiple nodules to diffuse lymphangiomatosis.[17] Most cases are microcystic or solid, and may show central scarring.[17]

Lymphangiomatosis may show multiorgan involvement, most frequently in the neck, mediastinum, axilla, or retroperitoneum.[32] The liver is the most common site of secondary involvement.[17] Diffuse lymphangiomatosis has the worst prognosis and may be life threatening, especially in children.[17,34] Takayama and colleagues[33] presented a rare case with presence of papillary endothelial proliferation and a pattern of scarlike fibrosis.

Lymphangiomas are usually an incidental finding in asymptomatic patients undergoing routine radiologic examination.[9] They may also present as a large, symptomatic mass as a result of compression of adjacent tissue.[32] The severity of symptoms, primarily left upper quadrant abdominal pain, is correlated with the size of the lesion.[35] This lesion can also present with a variety of complications, including portal hypertension, hemorrhage, coagulopathy, and hypersplenism.

Splenic lymphangiomas are slow-growing tumors that present primarily in childhood, but there are cases of detection in adults.[32] On MDCT, these lesions range from a few millimeters to several centimeters in diameter and are typically subcapsular in location.[17] Lesions appear as thin-walled, well-marginated masses with low-attenuation.[9] They lack significant enhancement with contrast media, which may hinder detection.[35] The cystic subtype may also present with curvilinear peripheral mural calcifications.[17] The spleen can appear mottled with poorly defined lesions both before and after contrast injection.[34] Lesions may also present with splenomegaly. Large, symptomatic lesions are generally treated with splenectomy, whereas small, solitary lymphangiomas are managed conservatively.[17]

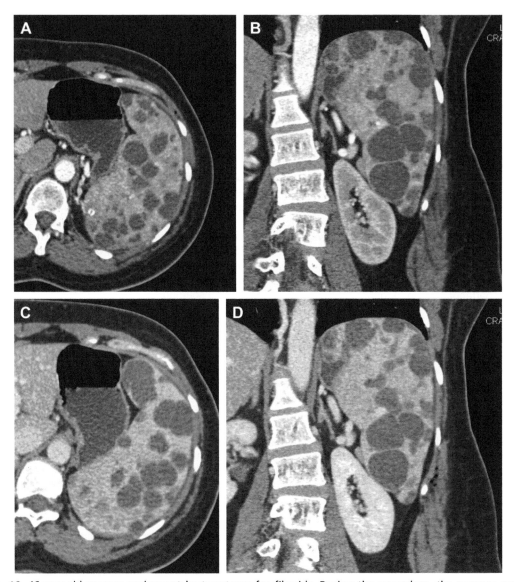

Fig. 16. 46-year-old woman underwent hysterectomy for fibroids. During the procedure, the surgeon noted splenomegaly and multiple splenic lesions. No biopsy was performed. Contrast-enhanced CT was performed in the arterial (A, B) and venous (C, D) phases and showed splenomegaly with multiple cystic lesions throughout the enlarged spleen. No enhancement of the lesions was noted. Hematologic work-up suggested that she had minimal residual splenic function. The patient now complained of mild pain. Splenectomy was performed and investigation revealed lymphangiomatosis.

Teaching point

Isolated splenic lymphangioma is uncommon in adults. These lesions typically are located subcapsularly and appear relatively cystic, without significant enhancement after IV contrast. Unless they are large and causing symptoms as a result of mass effect, they are not resected. Rarely, lymphangiomatosis can involve the spleen as well as other multiple other organs, such as the liver, nodes, and bones. Most splenic lymphangiomas are diagnosed in childhood.

Littoral Cell Angioma

A 59-year-old woman underwent CT for evaluation of incidental splenic lesions identified on an outside study (unavailable). The referring clinician reported that the patient had had known indeterminate splenic lesions for 5 years. No further clinical information was available. The CT shows multiple low-density splenic lesions varying in size (Fig. 17). The largest measured 6.5 cm. The remainder of the abdomen and pelvis were normal. The patient eventually underwent a splenectomy, which revealed multifocal littoral cell angioma.

Littoral cell angioma is a rare vascular neoplasm of the spleen first described in 1991.[36] It is commonly an incidental finding, although patients can sometimes present with anemia, thrombocytopenia, or splenomegaly.[37] Most littoral cell angiomas are benign, but there are case reports of malignant lesions.[17]

Teaching point
On CT, littoral cell angiomas usually appear as multiple low-density nodules varying in size up to 6 cm. They show enhancement after IV contrast and in some patients may become isodense to the spleen on delayed images. There is nothing specific about the CT appearance.

Splenic Infarct

A 74-year-old man with a history of alcohol abuse was admitted with multifocal pneumonia. A chest CT was ordered to evaluate the extent of the pneumonia (Fig. 18). Axial and contrast-enhanced CT showed a wedge-shaped low-density defect in the spleen compatible with infarct.

Splenic infarction can result from either arterial or venous compromise. Potential causes include hematologic disorders (sickle cell disease), thromboembolic disease (endocarditis, splenic vein thrombosis), vascular disorders (vasculitis),

and trauma. Most patients with splenic infarction are symptomatic, presenting with left upper quadrant pain and fever.[38] However, 30% to 50% of patients may have no symptoms, and therefore the radiologist may be the first to suggest the diagnosis.[38] The CT appearance varies depending on the acuity and cause. Initially infarcts may be hemorrhagic and as they heal they become fibrotic. They may resolve completely or leave a scar, which may calcify (see **Fig. 8**).

The classic CT appearance is a wedge-shaped area of decreased density, best seen on contrast-enhanced scans. Multiple lesions may be present. Acutely, the borders may be ill defined, but in the subacute phase, the borders are usually sharply demarcated. Air may sometimes be seen within the infarct as it heals (**Fig. 19**). Over time the wedge-shaped defect becomes smaller and resolves completely or results in a scar or calcification. In rare cases the entire spleen may undergo global infarction, resulting in only a thin rim of peripheral enhancement related to the capsule (**Fig. 20**).

Teaching point
In a busy clinical practice, it is likely you will encounter a patient with unsuspected splenic infraction. It is important not to misinterpret infarcts as masses or abscesses. Clinical history is helpful in determining potential embolic cause, including a history of endocarditis. In addition, the presence of other infarcts, in the kidneys for

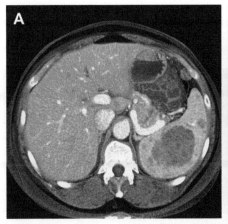
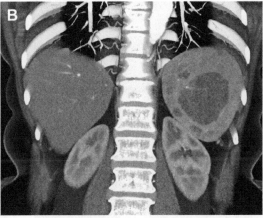

Fig. 17. 59-year-old woman underwent CT for evaluation of incidental splenic lesions identified on an outside study (unavailable). The referring clinician reported that the patient had had known indeterminate splenic lesions for 5 years. No further clinical information was available. (*A*) Axial and (*B*) coronal contrast-enhanced CT shows multiple low-density splenic lesions varying in size. The largest measured 6.5 cm. The remainder of the abdomen and pelvis were normal. The patient eventually underwent a splenectomy, which revealed multifocal littoral cell angioma.

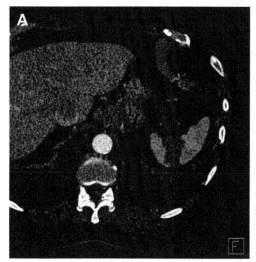 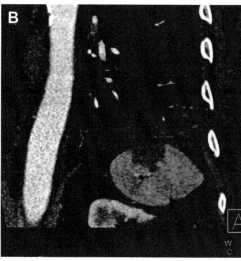

Fig. 18. 74-year-old man with history of alcohol abuse was admitted with multifocal pneumonia. A chest CT was ordered to evaluate the extent of the pneumonia (see Fig. 17). (*A*) Axial and (*B*) contrast-enhanced CT shows a wedge-shaped low-density defect in the spleen compatible with infarct.

example, can help support the diagnosis. A careful assessment of the splenic vasculature helps identify other potential causes such as vasculitis or splenic vein thrombosis.

Isolated Splenic Lesions in Patients with Known Malignancy

A 47 year-old woman underwent a chest CT for the evaluation of chest pain (Fig. 21). Contrast-enhanced chest CT showed a 5-cm anterior mediastinal mass and an 8-mm isolated low-density splenic lesion. The remainder of the chest, abdomen, and pelvis were unremarkable. The splenic lesion measured 8 mm in diameter and 57 HU on the contrast-enhanced scan. Noncontrast images were not obtained. There were no previous studies for comparison. Based on the CT appearance of the mediastinal mass and the clinical history, thymoma was the leading diagnosis. The radiologist stated that the isolated splenic lesion was "most likely benign."

The patient underwent thoracotomy and investigation revealed a pathologic stage-II (T2 N0) thymoma. The thymoma was completely encapsulated on gross examination with microscopic foci of invasion into

Fig. 19. 25-year-old man underwent splenic artery embolization after a traumatic injury. 5 days later the patient developed a fever. A contrast-enhanced CT shows embolization coils. There is a large splenic infarct with air.

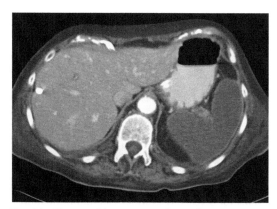

Fig. 20. 69-year-old woman 5 days after cystectomy for bladder cancer developed hypotension and sepsis. Contrast-enhanced CT shows global splenic infarction.

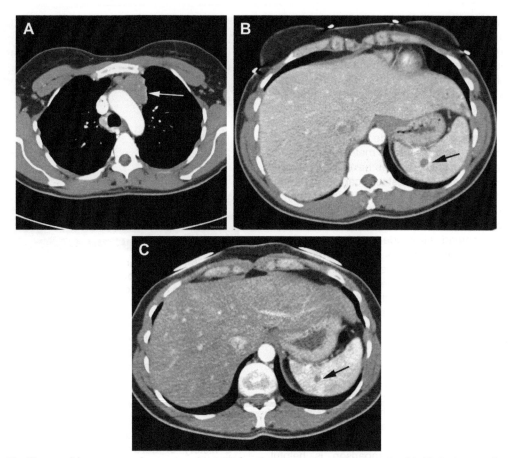

Fig. 21. 47-year-old woman underwent a chest CT for the evaluation of chest pain. (*A, B*) Contrast-enhanced chest CT showed a 5-cm anterior mediastinal mass and an 8-mm isolated low-density splenic lesion. The remainder of the chest, abdomen, and pelvis were unremarkable. The splenic lesion measured 57 HU on the contrast-enhanced scan. Based on the CT appearance of the mediastinal mass and the clinical history, thymoma was the leading diagnosis. The radiologist stated that the isolated splenic lesion was "most likely benign." The patient underwent thoracotomy and investigation revealed a pathologic stage-II (T2 N0) thymoma. The thymoma was completely encapsulated on gross examination with microscopic foci of invasion into the mediastinal adipose tissue. The patient also underwent adjuvant radiation. A follow-up CT 2 years later shows the splenic lesion to be unchanged in size and appearance (*C*).

the mediastinal adipose tissue. The patient also underwent adjuvant radiation. A follow-up CT 2 years later showed the splenic lesion to be unchanged in size and appearance.

This patient scenario is routinely encountered in practice. Isolated splenic lesions (one or more) are noted in a patient with suspected or known malignancy. What is the likelihood that these lesions represent splenic metastases without evidence of other sites of metastases?

Although the spleen is the largest organ in the reticuloendothelial system (RES), it is an uncommon site for metastases. The spleen is only the 10th most common site of metastases.[39] In an autopsy series conducted over a 10-year period, Rane and colleagues[40] reported only a 1.45% incidence of splenic involvement by neoplasms. The investigators noted that isolated splenic metastases are uncommon. Typically when metastases were noted in the spleen, multiple other organs were also involved. The reason for the uncommon occurrence of splenic metastases may be the lack of afferent lymphatics in the spleen.[39]

In another autopsy series by Schon and colleagues,[41] investigators analyzed 8563 autopsy files from 1980 to 1999. In 1898 cases a solid malignancy was noted; these included 1774 carcinomas, 36 sarcomas, and 27 malignant melanomas. Metastases to the spleen occurred in 3% of cases.[41] The most frequent primary tumors with splenic metastases were lung cancer, melanoma, and breast cancer (Fig. 22). Patients with testicular germ cell tumors, malignant melanoma, and small-cell lung cancer had the highest frequency of splenic involvement. In this study, most metastases were detected macroscopically (48/57).[41] Kaposi sarcoma in patients with AIDS can commonly involve the spleen, but there is always disseminated disease outside the spleen (Fig. 23).

Therefore, isolated splenic metastases are rare. Only approximately 40 cases have been reported in the literature.[42–44] Metastases can occur through hematogenous spread via the splenic artery, or rarely spread through the splenic vein in patients with portal hypertension. It is also possible for the tumor to spread retrograde from lymph nodes in the splenic hilum. Implants on the surface of the spleen are seen in patients with carcinomatosis from ovarian cancer, adenocarcinoma of the gastrointestinal tract, and pancreatic cancer. Direct tumor invasion of the spleen is also possible, usually from adjacent tumors in the pancreatic tail, stomach, or left kidney.

Teaching point
Isolated splenic metastases in patients with known or suspected malignancies are extremely uncommon. Therefore if there are no signs of metastases in other organs, isolated splenic lesions detected on CT are likely benign. If there are old studies, then comparison is helpful. However, in the absence of comparison studies, these lesions should be presumed benign. If there is something about the lesion that is suspicious,

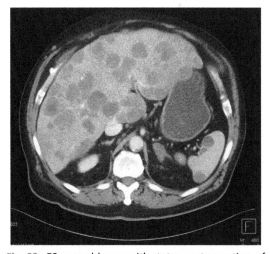

Fig. 22. 58-year-old man with status post resection of deep melanoma from his back with a high mitotic rate and 11/22 positive nodes. Contrast-enhanced CT shows widespread metastases in the liver and spleen. The scan 3 months previously (not shown) showed no evidence of metastatic disease.

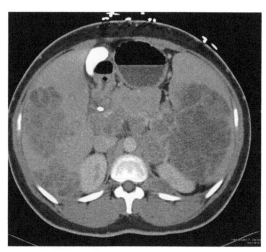

Fig. 23. 26-year-old man with AIDS and disseminated Kaposi sarcoma. CT shows a large splenic metastasis. Metastases are also noted in the liver and retroperitoneal nodes.

then in select cases a positron emission tomography (PET) scan or biopsy may be useful. However, in our practice this action is almost never necessary.

Sarcoidosis

A 41-year-old African American woman, with a history of borderline hypertension for 2 years, presented to the emergency department complaining of chest pain. A chest CT was performed and revealed multiple low-density splenic lesions (Fig. 24). The radiologist suggested the possibility of sarcoid. Bronchoscopy was performed and biopsy revealed noncaseating granuloma, compatible with sarcoid.

Sarcoidosis is a systemic disorder of unknown cause that typically presents with noncaseating granulomas and proliferation of epithelioid cells at numerous sites, primarily the lungs (90% of cases).[45] Splenic involvement is common, with a prevalence of 24% to 59% on needle biopsy in patients with known disease.[46] Splenic involvement may be associated with liver involvement (Fig. 25). However, isolated splenic disease is rare and most patients with splenic involvement are asymptomatic without any signs of organ dysfunction.[46] Symptomatic patients (2% of cases), usually with massive splenomegaly, may present with fever, weight loss, reduced appetite, and/or abdominal pain.[47] Asymptomatic patients, with or without mild splenomegaly, do not require any therapeutic intervention, but should be monitored for rare complications. Most symptomatic

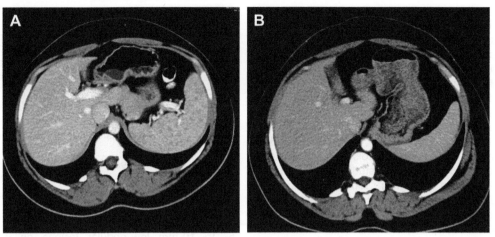

Fig. 24. 41-year-old African American woman, with a history of borderline hypertension for the last 2 years, presented to the emergency department complaining of chest pain. A chest CT was performed and revealed multiple low-density splenic lesions (*A*). The radiologist suggested the possibility of sarcoid. Bronchoscopy was performed and biopsy revealed noncaseating granuloma, compatible with sarcoid. (*B*) Follow-up CT 2 years later shows resolution of the previously noted splenic lesions.

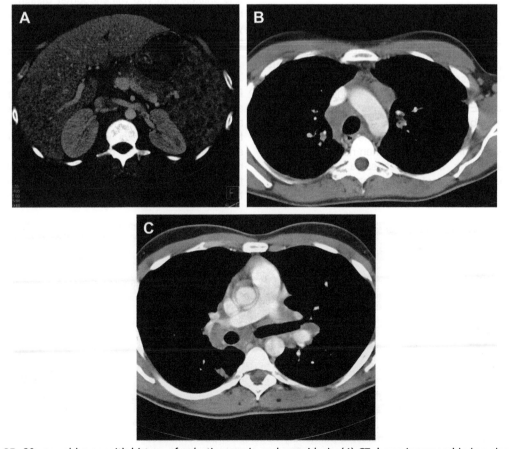

Fig. 25. 29-year-old man with history of aplastic anemia and sarcoidosis. (*A*) CT shows innumerable low-density lesions in the liver and spleen along with portal adenopathy. (*B*, *C*) Chest CT shows mediastinal and hilar adenopathy.

patients respond well to corticosteroid therapy. Splenectomy is a viable option in patients with substantial splenomegaly who fail drug therapy and show severe complications, including hematological abnormalities.[47]

Splenic involvement in sarcoidosis is usually an incidental finding on radiologic examination. Hypodense nodules, without peripheral enhancement, appear on contrast-enhanced CT scans of the spleen.[48] The differential diagnosis includes lymphoma, diffuse metastatic disease, and granulomatous infection (Fig. 26). A study of 32 patients by Warshauer and colleagues[46] reported adenopathy on CT in 76% of cases, most commonly at the porta hepatis and paraaortic region. All patients in this study had multiple splenic nodules, with a mean size of 0.9 cm (range, 0.3–2.0 cm), and 17 patients also presented with hepatic lesions of similar dimensions.[46] Splenic sarcoidosis may also appear as a necrotic mass with punctate calcifications, as reported in 16% of patients in one study.[49]

Teaching point

We see this scenario a few times each year. A young or middle-aged woman undergoes a CT for vague symptoms. The radiologist reports multiple low-density splenic lesions, suspicious for metastases. The patient undergoes an extensive work-up to search for a primary site of disease. Eventually the diagnosis is made after a splenic biopsy or biopsy of mediastinal/hilar nodes. Consider sarcoidosis as the cause of isolated splenic lesions, especially when noted as an incidental finding. In some cases, a chest CT may be indicated to look for adenopathy, which then can be biopsied to confirm the diagnosis.

OTHER TOPICS
Disseminated Infection to the Spleen

A variety of infections can spread hematogenously, resulting in hepatic and splenic abscesses or microabscesses. However, splenic disease without hepatic involvement is rare. Also it is uncommon to have these infections diagnosed as incidental findings, because patients usually present with fever, chills abdominal pain, nausea, and vomiting.[7]

Immunocompromised individuals are prone to disseminated fungal infection.[7] *Candida* is the most frequently encountered, followed by *Aspergillus*, *Cryptococcus*, and histoplasmosis.

CT fungal microabscesses appear as multiple 5- to 10-mm low-nodular lesions on venous phase imaging (Fig. 27). Sometimes ring enhancement is noted on arterial phase images. The lesions can appear cystic. Liver and splenic involvement is typical. The kidneys may also be involved.

Teaching point

It is unlikely that you will encounter disseminated infection of the spleen as an incidental finding. If you do, there is almost certainly involvement of the liver and possibly kidney.

Peliosis

Peliosis is a rare condition most commonly affecting the liver, but occasionally involving the spleen. The cause is not definitely known, but there are associations with various conditions such as infections, use of anabolic steroids, and hematologic malignancies. Isolated peliosis of the spleen is rare.[50] Patients are usually asymptomatic and therefore peliosis may be an

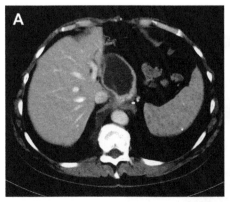
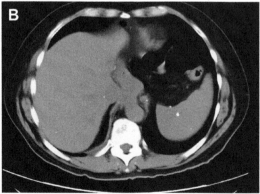

Fig. 26. 63-year-old man, 7.5 years after esophagectomy for adenocarcinoma. Patient underwent chest CT for follow-up of an incidentally detected pulmonary nodule. Contrast-enhanced CT showed multiple low-density splenic lesions (A). Only previous noncontrast CTs were available for comparison and showed punctate calcifications in the spleen (B). The radiologist was concerned about metastatic disease or lymphoma, so splenectomy was performed. Investigation revealed sarcoidosis.

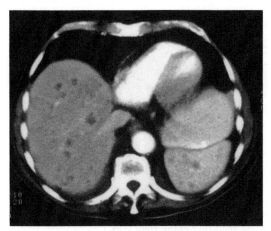

Fig. 27. AIDS. Contrast-enhanced CT shows numerous low-density lesions in the liver and spleen compatible with disseminated *Candida* infection.

incidental finding on CT or at autopsy. However, spontaneous splenic rupture has been reported.[51] Pathologically, peliosis is characterized by dilated sinusoids along with the formation of fluid-filled and blood-filled cavities within the splenic parenchyma.[52]

On contrast-enhanced CT, splenic peliosis appears as multiple small well-defined low-density or cystic lesions[51] (Fig. 28). The lesions may vary in size. Some lesions may appear hyperdense related to hemorrhage, and sometimes fluid/fluid levels may be apparent, related to the hematocrit effect. Various patterns of enhancement have been reported including early peripheral enhancement with delayed centripetal enhancement.

Teaching point
Isolated splenic peliosis is rare but should be considered in the right clinical setting when

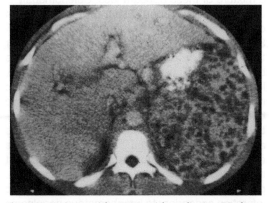

Fig. 28. Patient with AIDS with peliosis. CT shows multiple low-density splenic lesions. The liver was also involved. (*Courtesy of* Kyunghee Cho, MD, New York University-Langone Medical Center, New York.)

multiple hemorrhagic splenic lesions are noted, especially when associated with liver lesions.

PRIMARY SPLENIC MALIGNANCIES

Primary splenic malignancies are almost never incidentalomas. Patients are symptomatic. However, for completeness sake this topic is reviewed in the next section.

Angiosarcoma

Angiosarcoma of the spleen typically presents in patients more than 40 years of age, with no gender predilection.[17] Lesions are rarely discovered incidentally on radiologic examination. More commonly, patients are symptomatic, and some present with acute abdominal symptoms secondary to rupture.[53] Patients may also present with constitutional symptoms of fever, fatigue, and weight loss. Anemia, thrombocytopenia, or other coagulopathies are possible complications.

Although its incidence is low, primary angiosarcoma is the most common malignant nonlymphoid neoplasm of the spleen.[17,54] It is derived from the endothelium of splenic sinuses and manifests as disorganized anastomosing vascular channels lined by hyperchromatic, rapidly proliferating endothelial cells.[55] Diffuse involvement of the splenic parenchyma is commonly seen on pathologic examination, but some cases may also present as solitary lesions containing areas of hemorrhage and necrosis.[17] It is an extremely aggressive tumor, with less than 20% survival at 6 months after diagnosis. Approximately 70% of cases metastasize to the liver.[17] Other common sites of involvement include the lungs, bone, bone marrow, and lymphatic system.[6,17] Several case reports show associations with previous chemotherapy for lymphoma, radiation therapy for breast cancer, and thorotrast exposure.[17,54] The primary complication, present in one-third of cases, is spontaneous rupture of the lesion.

Splenomegaly is a common finding and lesions show an aggressive growth pattern, commonly presenting with metastatic disease at time of diagnosis.[17] On spiral CT scans, tumors appear as ill-defined splenic masses, which may show immediate focal enhancement with progressive centripetal enhancement (Fig. 29).[53] Splenic angiosarcoma often presents as multiple nodules of varying sizes on MDCT, but may also appear as a solitary mass of cystic and solid regions.[54] Nonenhanced images generally show hypoattenuating lesions with focal areas of high CT attenuation at sites of acute hemorrhage or hemosiderin deposits (Fig. 30).[9] Patients with thorotrast-induced disease may show high attenuation of

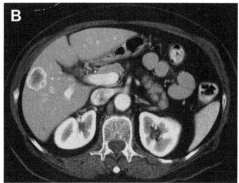

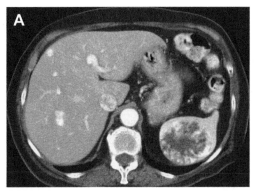

Fig. 29. 72-year-old woman with left upper quadrant pain. Contrast-enhanced CT shows a vascular enhancing splenic lesion (*A*) as well as enhancing liver lesions (*A, B*) compatible with metastatic splenic angiosarcoma. (*Courtesy of* Kyunghee Cho, MD, New York University-Langone Medical Center, New York.)

the liver or characteristic increased density of the spleen and lymph nodes.[9] Areas of punctate calcifications or massive calcification in a radial pattern have also been reported on CT.[56]

Teaching point

It is unlikely that you will encounter a splenic angiosarcoma as an incidental finding on CT. However, angiosarcoma should be given consideration when a splenic lesion with hemorrhage or unusual calcification is encountered, especially if there are associated vascular liver lesions.

Lymphoma

Lymphomatous involvement of the spleen is rarely an incidental finding. However, some patients may present with left upper quadrant abdominal fullness and pain, usually as a result of splenomegaly.[57] Nonspecific, systemic symptoms, including weight loss, malaise, and fever, are also noted in some cases and may prompt a CT.[12,57]

Lymphoma involves the spleen in both Hodgkin and non-Hodgkin subtypes and is currently the

most common malignant neoplasm of the spleen.[9] In most cases, it is a manifestation of systemic disease, and less than 2% of all lymphomas present as a primary, isolated splenic lesion.[9,12] Usually non-Hodgkin in type, primary splenic lymphomas are more common in older patients (mean age of 55 years) and in AIDS-related cases.[12,54] In patients with newly diagnosed, previously untreated disease, staging laparotomy revealed clinically unsuspected involvement of the spleen in approximately one-third of cases.[53] Hodgkin lymphoma presents with splenic lesions in 23% to 34% of patients, whereas non-Hodgkin lymphoma involves the spleen in 30% to 40% of cases during initial assessment.[9] Reported accuracies of CT for identifying splenic lymphomas range from 37% to 91%.[58]

Splenic involvement in lymphoma may present on MDCT as a homogeneous enlargement without masses, multiple milliary nodules (<1 cm), multiple lesions (usually >1 cm and <10 cm), or a single solitary mass (Fig. 31).[9] It may also present as a mixture of these appearances. Splenomegaly is a common finding on CT, but up to one-third of cases may present with normal-sized spleen.[53] Solitary and multifocal lesions measuring greater than 1 cm in diameter are easily detectable by CT and usually appear as discrete, low-attenuating masses[9,12] (Fig. 32). Splenic lymphomas are best characterized after a dynamic bolus of iodinated contrast material, which selectively increases the attenuation of normal hepatic and splenic parenchyma.[58] Primary lymphomas are usually confined to the splenic capsule, but may also involve the diaphragm, stomach, pancreas, and/or abdominal wall. Cases of splenic infarction secondary to lymphomatous neoplasms appear as peripheral, wedge-shaped lesions of low attenuation. Calcification may be observed in aggressive lesions and after therapy.[9,58]

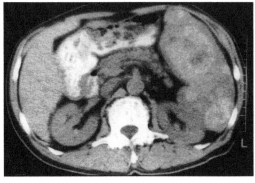

Fig. 30. Noncontrast CT in a patient with angiosarcoma shows multiple splenic lesions with hemorrhage.

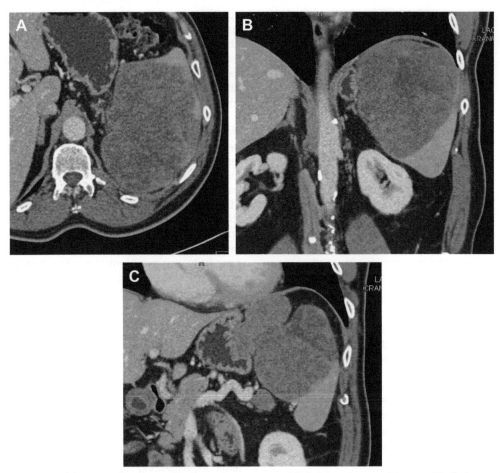

Fig. 31. 64-year-old man underwent a CT after minor trauma. (A) Axial and coronal images (B, C) show a large low-density splenic mass. There is associated adenopathy (best seen *in* C). No other sites of disease were noted. Splenectomy was performed and shows diffuse B-cell lymphoma.

Teaching point

You are unlikely to encounter a splenic lymphoma as an incidental finding. However, it may be seen in patients presenting with vague symptoms. Most cases of lymphomatous splenic involvement have other sites of disease and associated adenopathy, which aid in the diagnosis. Isolated primary splenic lymphoma represents less than 2 % of all lymphomas. Additional imaging or biopsy may be needed in these cases.

Splenic Biopsy

Fine-needle aspiration biopsy and core biopsy are of considerable diagnostic value after incidental detection of a suspicious splenic lesion on contrast-enhanced CT. Image-guided percutaneous splenic interventions can be performed safely with minimal risk of complications. Several studies have shown the usefulness and safety of splenic biopsy in assessing incidentalomas. In

one such study, Lucey and colleagues[59] retrospectively analyzed 24 splenic biopsies, 19 with sonographic guidance and 5 with CT guidance, performed after detection of an uncharacterized lesion on contrast-enhanced CT (12 incidentalomas). Thirteen patients underwent fine-needle aspiration biopsy only, 3 underwent core biopsy only, and 8 underwent both procedures. These investigators reported a diagnostic success rate of 91%, with only 3 cases of complications, including one minor intraabdominal bleed and 2 large areas of perisplenic bleeding. Other recent studies have reported success rates of splenic biopsy ranging from 63% to 89%, with complication rates ranging from 1.5% to 13%.[60–64] The most common complication is bleeding, which may not require any intervention in minor cases, but splenectomy is usually indicated in hemodynamically unstable patients. Rates of hemorrhage range from 0% to 2% in recent series and usually result from biopsy of vascular lesions,

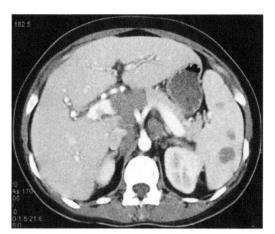

Fig. 32. Patient with B-cell lymphoma. Contrast-enhanced CT shows multiple low-density splenic lesions associated with extensive adenopathy.

such as littoral cell angioma and angiosarcoma.[59] Core-needle biopsy generally increases the risk of significant hemorrhage.

Percutaneous fluid aspiration can also be useful for diagnosis of incidentally discovered splenic fluid density lesions. This procedure is usually indicated in febrile patients with low-attenuating splenic lesions on CT. It may be performed to differentiate among a splenic cyst, an infarct, and an abscess. Ultrasound- (US-) and CT-guided fluid aspiration procedures were shown to have a high diagnostic success rate, with minimal complications in a recent study.[59]

Teaching point

Biopsy of splenic lesions is relatively safe, but is usually not necessary. Biopsy of splenic lesions is necessary only in rare patient scenarios, usually involving certain patient populations or because of the potentially life-threatening nature of some lesions, such as splenic abscess or angiosarcoma.

THE ROLE OF PET AND OTHER MODALITIES

Given that most incidentally detected splenic lesions are benign, performing invasive diagnostic procedures on all incidentalomas may be over-treatment. However, splenic abnormalities on CT in certain patient populations cannot be ignored because of the potentially life-threatening nature of some lesions. Therefore, noninvasive imaging modalities, including PET, US, and magnetic resonance (MR) imaging, can be useful in selecting high-risk patients for splenic biopsy to a make definitive diagnosis.

Incidental splenic lesions can be further evaluated for malignancy with [18F]fluorodeoxyglucose (FDG)-PET and hybrid PET/CT. Solid malignancies of the spleen are expected to show abnormal

uptake patterns of FDG, whereas some benign lesions, like splenic abscesses, may also show abnormalities on imaging leading to false-positive results. Granulomatous diseases, like tuberculosis, and inflammatory pseudotumors can show abnormal uptake of FDG to mimic patterns of malignancy.

In a recent study, Mester and colleagues[63] showed that FDG-PET/CT can reliably differentiate between benign and malignant solid splenic lesions in patients with known malignant diseases, including lymphoma, lung cancer, melanoma, and gastrointestinal and gynecologic malignancies. FDG-PET/CT was also shown to be effective in following up patients with incidentally discovered splenic lesions on conventional imaging modalities, like contrast-enhanced CT. The sensitivity, specificity, positive predictive value, and negative predictive value of FDG-PET/CT in differentiating benign from solid, malignant splenic incidentalomas were 100%, 83%, 80%, and 100%, respectively.[63] However, caution should be taken to avoid false-negative results, especially in non-FDG–avid tumors, like renal cell carcinomas or thyroid cancers, which may metastasize to the spleen.

Contrast-enhanced ultrasonography (CEUS) may also be used for further evaluation of incidentally detected splenic lesions and allows for accurate characterization of size and shape of the spleen. Limitations of this modality include problems in visualizing deep pole and subphrenic areas, and shadowing from the left colonic flexure.[65]

In a prospective study of 35 patients, von Herbay and colleagues[66] showed the ability of low-mechanical-index CEUS to differentiate between benign and malignant lesions of the spleen. These investigators used a second-generation micro-bubble contrast agent that allows for continuous real-time imaging and dynamic analysis of enhancement patterns in the early phase, which is critical for diagnosis. A combination of homogeneous contrast enhancement in the early phase and rapid washout and demarcation in the parenchymal phase (60 seconds after injection) indicated splenic malignancy.[66] In contrast, benign lesions showed clear demarcation in both the early and parenchymal phases of CEUS. Stang and colleagues[67] showed that a progressively hypoenhancing lesion was 87% positively predictive and 100% sensitive for malignancy, but only 83% specific. A constantly nonenhancing or isoenhancing lesion was 100% positively predictive for benign disease. Compared with unenhanced sonography, CEUS improves diagnostic accuracy by 17% to 38%.

Contrast-enhanced MR imaging of the spleen may also supplement findings on CT. Gadolinium-based contrast agents and RES-targeted superparamagnetic iron oxide particles are both used for characterization of splenic lesions.[68] Dynamic imaging after injection of contrast media provides information about vascularity and visualization of characteristic filling patterns to guide diagnosis. In addition, RES-specific contrast media may be used to identify accessory splenic tissue and abdominal or intra-thoracic splenosis.[69]

SUMMARY

Incidentalomas of the spleen are not uncommon in a busy practice. Most isolated splenic lesions are benign and are of no clinical significance. However, it is important that the radiologist is familiar with the characteristic CT appearance of a wide range of splenic disease conditions. Also comparison with old scans is always helpful, as is correlation with relevant clinical information.

REFERENCES

1. Ekeh AP, Walusimbi M, Brigham E, et al. The prevalence of incidental findings on abdominal computed tomography scans of trauma patients. J Emerg Med 2010;38(4):484–9.
2. Paluska TR, Sise MJ, Sack DI, et al. Incidental CT findings in trauma patients: incidence and implications for care of the injured. J Trauma 2007;62:157–61.
3. Brennan TV, Lipshutz GS, Posselt AM, et al. Congenital cleft spleen with CT scan appearance of high-grade splenic laceration after blunt abdominal trauma. J Emerg Med 2003;25:139–42.
4. Gayer G, Zissin R, Apter S, et al. CT findings in congenital anomalies of the spleen. Br J Radiol 2001;74:767–72.
5. Toure L, Bedard J, Sawan B, et al. Case note: intra-pancreatic accessory spleen mimicking a pancreatic endocrine tumour. Can J Surg 2010;53:E1–2.
6. Freeman JL, Jafri SZ, Roberts JL, et al. CT of congenital and acquired abnormalities of the spleen. Radiographics 1993;13:597–610.
7. Bean MJ, Horton KM, Fishman EK. Concurrent focal hepatic and splenic lesions: a pictorial guide to differential diagnosis. J Comput Assist Tomogr 2004;28:605–12.
8. Reeders JW, Yee J, Gore RM, et al. Gastrointestinal infection in the immunocompromised (AIDS) patient. Eur Radiol 2004;14(Suppl 3):E84–102.
9. Rabushka LS, Kawashima A, Fishman EK. Imaging of the spleen: CT with supplemental MR examination. Radiographics 1994;14:307–32.
10. Tsakayannis DE, Mitchell K, Kozakewich HP, et al. Splenic preservation in the management of splenic epidermoid cysts in children. J Pediatr Surg 1995; 30:1468–70.
11. Hansen MB, Moller AC. Splenic cysts. Surg Laparosc Endosc Percutan Tech 2004;14:316–22.
12. Urrutia M, Mergo PJ, Ros LH, et al. Cystic masses of the spleen: radiologic-pathologic correlation. Radiographics 1996;16:107–29.
13. Dawes LG, Malangoni MA. Cystic masses of the spleen. Am Surg 1986;52:333–6.
14. Franquet T, Montes M, Lecumberri FJ, et al. Hydatid disease of the spleen: imaging findings in nine patients. AJR Am J Roentgenol 1990;154:525–8.
15. von Sinner WN, Stridbeck H. Hydatid disease of the spleen. Ultrasonography, CT and MR imaging. Acta Radiol 1992;33:459–61.
16. Ros PR, Moser RP Jr, Dachman AH, et al. Hemangioma of the spleen: radiologic-pathologic correlation in ten cases. Radiology 1987;162:73–7.
17. Abbott RM, Levy AD, Aguilera NS, et al. From the archives of the AFIP: primary vascular neoplasms of the spleen: radiologic-pathologic correlation. Radiographics 2004;24:1137–63.
18. Elsayes KM, Narra VR, Mukundan G, et al. MR imaging of the spleen: spectrum of abnormalities. Radiographics 2005;25:967–82.
19. Disler DG, Chew FS. Splenic hemangioma. AJR Am J Roentgenol 1991;157:44.
20. Moss CN, Van Dyke JA, Koehler RE, et al. Multiple cavernous hemangiomas of the spleen: CT findings. J Comput Assist Tomogr 1986;10:338–40.
21. Warshauer DM, Molina PL, Worawattanakul S. The spotted spleen: CT and clinical correlation in a tertiary care center. J Comput Assist Tomogr 1998;22:694–702.
22. Ramani M, Reinhold C, Semelka RC, et al. Splenic hemangiomas and hamartomas: MR imaging characteristics of 28 lesions. Radiology 1997;202: 166–72.
23. Ferrozzi F, Bova D, Draghi F, et al. CT findings in primary vascular tumors of the spleen. AJR Am J Roentgenol 1996;166:1097–101.
24. Willcox TM, Speer RW, Schlinkert RT, et al. Hemangioma of the spleen: presentation, diagnosis, and management. J Gastrointest Surg 2000;4:611–3.
25. Falk S, Stutte HJ. Hamartomas of the spleen: a study of 20 biopsy cases. Histopathology 1989; 14:603–12.
26. Krishnan J, Frizzera G. Two splenic lesions in need of clarification: hamartoma and inflammatory pseudotumor. Semin Diagn Pathol 2003;20:94–104.
27. Conlon S, Royston D, Murphy P. Splenic hamartoma. Cytopathology 2007;18:200–2.
28. Yoshizawa J, Mizuno R, Yoshida T, et al. Spontaneous rupture of splenic hamartoma: a case report. J Pediatr Surg 1999;34:498–9.

29. Lam KY, Yip KH, Peh WC. Splenic vascular lesions: unusual features and a review of the literature. Aust N Z J Surg 1999;69:422–5.

30. Ohtomo K, Fukuda H, Mori K, et al. CT and MR appearances of splenic hamartoma. J Comput Assist Tomogr 1992;16:425–8.

31. Contini S, Corradi D. Hand-assisted laparoscopic splenectomy for a splenic hamartoma. Surg Endosc 2002;16:871.

32. Solomou EG, Patriarheas GV, Mpadra FA, et al. Asymptomatic adult cystic lymphangioma of the spleen: case report and review of the literature. Magn Reson Imaging 2003;21:81–4.

33. Takayama A, Nakashima O, Kobayashi K, et al. Splenic lymphangioma with papillary endothelial proliferation: a case report and review of the literature. Pathol Int 2003;53:483–8.

34. Wadsworth DT, Newman B, Abramson SJ, et al. Splenic lymphangiomatosis in children. Radiology 1997;202:173–6.

35. Komatsuda T, Ishida H, Konno K, et al. Splenic lymphangioma: US and CT diagnosis and clinical manifestations. Abdom Imaging 1999;24:414–7.

36. Falk S, Stutte HJ, Frizzera G. Littoral cell angioma. A novel splenic vascular lesion demonstrating histiocytic differentiation. Am J Surg Pathol 1991;15:1023–33.

37. Bhatt S, Huang J, Dogra V. Littoral cell angioma of the spleen. AJR Am J Roentgenol 2007;188:1365–6.

38. Nores M, Phillips EH, Morgenstern L, et al. The clinical spectrum of splenic infarction. Am Surg 1998;64:182–8.

39. Berge T. Splenic metastases. Frequencies and patterns. Acta Pathol Microbiol Scand A 1974;82:499–506.

40. Rane SR, Bagwan IN, Pingle P, et al. Splenic tumours–autopsy study of ten years. Indian J Pathol Microbiol 2005;48:186–9.

41. Schon CA, Gorg C, Ramaswamy A, et al. Splenic metastases in a large unselected autopsy series. Pathol Res Pract 2006;202:351–6.

42. Lam KY, Tang V. Metastatic tumors to the spleen: a 25-year clinicopathologic study. Arch Pathol Lab Med 2000;124:526–30.

43. Klein B, Stein M, Kuten A, et al. Splenomegaly and solitary spleen metastasis in solid tumors. Cancer 1987;60:100–2.

44. Schmidt BJ, Smith SL. Isolated splenic metastasis from primary lung adenocarcinoma. South Med J 2004;97:298–300.

45. Zia H, Zemon H, Brody F. Laparoscopic splenectomy for isolated sarcoidosis of the spleen. J Laparoendosc Adv Surg Tech A 2005;15:160–2.

46. Warshauer DM, Molina PL, Hamman SM, et al. Nodular sarcoidosis of the liver and spleen: analysis of 32 cases. Radiology 1995;195:757–62.

47. Mihailovic-Vucinic V, Sharma OP. The spleen in sarcoidosis. In: Atlas of sarcoidosis. London: Springer; 2005. p. 65–7.

48. Warshauer DM, Semelka RC, Ascher SM. Nodular sarcoidosis of the liver and spleen: appearance on MR images. J Magn Reson Imaging 1994;4:553–7.

49. Folz SJ, Johnson CD, Swensen SJ. Abdominal manifestations of sarcoidosis in CT studies. J Comput Assist Tomogr 1995;19:573–9.

50. Tsokos M, Puschel K. Isolated peliosis of the spleen: report of 2 autopsy cases. Am J Forensic Med Pathol 2004;25:251–4.

51. Lashbrook DJ, James RW, Phillips AJ, et al. Splenic peliosis with spontaneous splenic rupture: report of two cases. BMC Surg 2006;6:9.

52. Tsokos M, Erbersdobler A. Pathology of peliosis. Forensic Sci Int 2005;149:25–33.

53. Kawamoto S, Fishman EK. MDCT evaluation of the spleen. In: Fishman EK, Jeffrey RB Jr, editors. Multidetector CT: principles, techniques, clinical applications. Philadelphia: Lippincott Williams & Williams; 2004. p. 255–69.

54. Warshauer DM, Hall HL. Solitary splenic lesions. Semin Ultrasound CT MR 2006;27:370–88.

55. Takato H, Iwamoto H, Ikezu M, et al. Splenic hemangiosarcoma with sinus endothelial differentiation. Acta Pathol Jpn 1993;43:702–8.

56. Kinoshita T, Ishii K, Yajima Y, et al. Splenic hemangiosarcoma with massive calcification. Abdom Imaging 1999;24:185–7.

57. Castellino RA, Hoppe RT, Blank N, et al. Computed tomography, lymphography, and staging laparotomy: correlations in initial staging of Hodgkin disease. AJR Am J Roentgenol 1984;143:37–41.

58. Thomas JL, Bernardino ME, Vermess M, et al. EOE-13 in the detection of hepatosplenic lymphoma. Radiology 1982;145:629–34.

59. Lucey BC, Boland GW, Maher MM, et al. Percutaneous nonvascular splenic intervention: a 10-year review. AJR Am J Roentgenol 2002;179:1591–6.

60. Keogan MT, Freed KS, Paulson EK, et al. Imaging-guided percutaneous biopsy of focal splenic lesions: update on safety and effectiveness. AJR Am J Roentgenol 1999;172:933–7.

61. Caraway NP, Fanning CV. Use of fine-needle aspiration biopsy in the evaluation of splenic lesions in a cancer center. Diagn Cytopathol 1997;16:312–6.

62. Venkataramu NK, Gupta S, Sood BP, et al. Ultrasound guided fine needle aspiration biopsy of splenic lesions. Br J Radiol 1999;72:953–6.

63. Metser U, Miller E, Kessler A, et al. Solid splenic masses: evaluation with 18F-FDG PET/CT. J Nucl Med 2005;46:52–9.

64. Metser U, Even-Sapir E. The role of 18F-FDG PET/CT in the evaluation of solid splenic masses. Semin Ultrasound CT MR 2006;27:420–5.

65. Catalano O, Sandomenico F, Vallone P, et al. Contrast-enhanced sonography of the spleen. Semin Ultrasound CT MR 2006;27:426–33.

66. von Herbay A, Barreiros AP, Ignee A, et al. Contrast-enhanced ultrasonography with SonoVue: differentiation between benign and malignant lesions of the spleen. J Ultrasound Med 2009;28:421–34.

67. Stang A, Keles H, Hentschke S, et al. Differentiation of benign from malignant focal splenic lesions using sulfur hexafluoride-filled microbubble contrast-enhanced pulse-inversion sonography. AJR Am J Roentgenol 2009;193:709–21.

68. Schneider G, Reimer P, Mamann A, et al. Contrast agents in abdominal imaging: current and future directions. Top Magn Reson Imaging 2005;16:107–24.

69. Berman AJ, Zahalsky MP, Okon SA, et al. Distinguishing splenosis from renal masses using ferumoxide-enhanced magnetic resonance imaging. Urology 2003;62:748.

The Incidental Pancreatic Cyst

Alec J. Megibow, MD, MPH[a],*, Mark E. Baker, MD[b],
Richard M. Gore, MD[c], Andrew Taylor, MD[d]

KEYWORDS

• Pancreatic cyst • Incidental finding • MRI
• MDCT • Management

The discovery of a pancreatic cyst in an asymptomatic patient presents an immediate challenge to the interpreting radiologist, the clinician who manages the patient, and patients themselves. The widespread use of multidetector row CT (MDCT) or MRI in an aging population has accelerated the discovery of these lesions.

The frequency of pancreatic cysts identified with CT scanning is reported to be between 290 of 24039 (1.2%)[1] and 73 of 2832 (2.6%).[2] For MRI, the reported frequency is significantly higher, at between 283 of 1444 (19.9%)[3] and 83 of 616 (13.5%).[4] Therefore, the practicing radiologist could anticipate seeing a pancreatic cyst anywhere from 1 to 2 or 14 to 20 times per 100 cases imaged. For some practices, this could be a daily occurrence.

Although for many years the most common pancreatic cyst was believed to be a pseudocyst, cystic pancreatic neoplasms, serous cystadenoma, mucinous cystic tumor (MCT), and intraductal papillary mucinous tumors (IPMTs) now account for most of the pancreatic cysts seen in asymptomatic individuals.[5] Cystic pancreatic tumors are most often benign or low-grade indolent neoplasms; however, if the cyst is mucinous (eg, intraductal papillary mucinous neoplasm or MCT), a variable but well-established malignant potential exists.[6,7] This variable malignant potential of these cysts is the source of discomfort for all clinicians. The relative inaccessibility of the pancreas (as opposed to colon, breast, or even lung) to easy biopsy further exacerbates the problem.

When a cyst is discovered on an imaging study in a patient without symptoms directly referable to the pancreas, the following questions are immediately raised: can the lesion be accurately diagnosed or is the appropriate management clear from the examination, is the best management approach to suggest watchful waiting with follow-up imaging, what is the best method for imaging follow-up, and what is the optimal frequency of follow-up?

CAN THE LESION EITHER BE ACCURATELY DIAGNOSED OR IS THE APPROPRIATE MANAGEMENT CLEAR FROM THE EXAMINATION?

Morphologic features that can be assessed through imaging, allowing cyst characterization, include presence or absence of septa/loculations, presence and location of calcification, location of the mass within the pancreas, and presence of main pancreatic duct involvement[8–11] (Fig. 1). Dense septa are predictive of a serous cystadenoma, although oligocystic (few or no septa) variants can be encountered.[12,13] A simple but useful classification system differentiates pancreatic cysts into four gross morphologic types based solely on imaging appearance at MDCT: (1) unilocular (pseudocysts, lymphoepithelial cysts, small IPMTs), (2) microcystic (serous cystadenoma), (3) macrocystic (mucinous cystic tumor, IPMTs), and (4) cysts with a solid component (solid pseudopapillary neoplasm, mucinous cystic neoplasm).[14] Overlap is anticipated in this classification, but

[a] Department of Radiology, New York University Langone Medical Center, New York, NY, USA
[b] Department of Radiology, Cleveland Clinic Foundation, Cleveland, OH, USA
[c] Department of Radiology, NorthShore University Health System, Pritzker School of Medicine, University of Chicago, 2650 Ridge Avenue, Evanston, IL, USA
[d] Department of Radiology, Virginia Commonwealth University Medical Center, Richmond, VA, USA
* Corresponding author.
E-mail address: alec.megibow@nyumc.org

Radiol Clin N Am 49 (2011) 349–359
doi:10.1016/j.rcl.2010.10.008

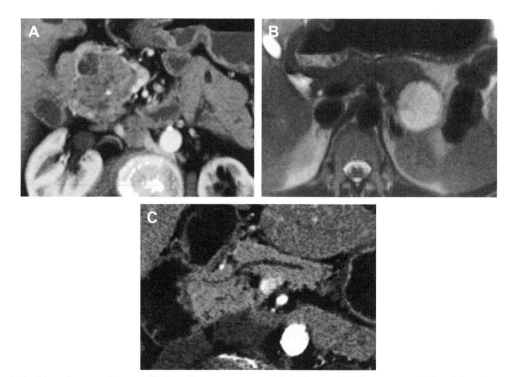

Fig. 1. Incidental cysts with specific imaging appearances. (*A*) The cyst in the pancreatic head has diagnostic features of a serous cystadenoma, including dense central septa, central calcification, and slightly larger peripheral cysts. (*B*) T2-weighted MRI shows a cyst in the pancreatic tail of a 50–year-old woman. The wall has slight lobulation, and a thin septum is present. These findings are typical of a mucinous cystic tumor (MCT). (*C*) A cyst was detected on the axial images; however, the volumetric MDCT data allow three-dimensional analysis, which enables detection of a neck connecting the cyst to the main pancreatic duct diagnostic of branch duct IPMT.

a likely diagnosis can be offered for most masses larger than 2 cm. Small cysts (<2 cm) will almost always appear unilocular regardless of origin.[15]

Serous cystadenoma is a benign lesion. Most can be described as either "honeycomb," "sponge-like," or oligocystic[8] depending on the density of septa. Because up to 5% of them can be either unilocular or contain few septa, the term *microcystic* is no longer used. Calcifications are present in approximately 30% of cases and are centrally located. Lobulation is frequent. Unusual appearances can be encountered, including obstructive dilatation of the main pancreatic duct, intratumoral hemorrhage, and a solid variant.[12,16]

Mucinous tumors are classified into two broad categories: parenchymal and intraductal. The latter is subdivided into tumors arising in the main duct, a side branch, or a combined (mixed) form. Parenchymal mucinous lesions, referred to as *MCTs*, can be suspected based when a cyst is present in the tail of the pancreas. They often will have at least one recognizable septum or are unilocular. They are most frequently encountered in perimenopausal women.[6] IPMTs or intraductal papillary mucinous neoplasms appear as

a dilated main pancreatic duct of variable length. Branch duct IPMT will have a visible communication with the MPD. Visualization of duct communication can be defined by three-dimensional imaging either with MRI/magnetic resonance cholangiopancreatography (MRCP) or MDCT.[17] They are seen more often in men.

Despite familiarity with the characteristic imaging features, many pancreatic cysts, particularly those smaller 2 cm in maximal diameter, are difficult if not impossible to specifically characterize (Fig. 2). Published studies comparing radiologic and surgical diagnosis of pancreatic cysts consistently reinforce the limitations of preoperative imaging diagnosis,[15,18] creating uncertainty for radiologists confronted with one of these lesions, because some will be benign and others will be low-grade neoplasms.

IS THE BEST MANAGEMENT APPROACH TO SUGGEST WATCHFUL WAITING WITH FOLLOW-UP IMAGING?

Most incidental pancreatic cysts are either benign or low-grade neoplasms. Among 61 asymptomatic

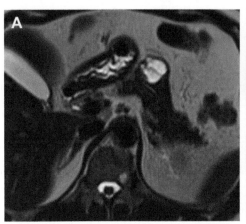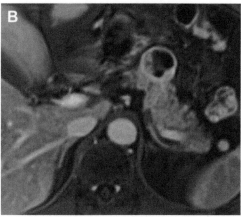

Fig. 2. Lack of specificity in the radiologic diagnosis of pancreatic cysts. (*A*) T2-weighted MR shows a septated cyst in pancreatic body. The appearance is compatible with MCT. (*B*) Gadolinium-enhanced image shows the cyst to have a thick wall, thick septum, and mural nodules. This appearance makes surgical removal advisable. The lesion was a neuroendocrine tumor.

patients in a cohort of 212 who had pancreatic cysts in whom operative correlation existed, 28% of asymptomatic cysts were mucinous cystic neoplasms, 27% were intraductal papillary mucinous neoplasms, 17% were serous cystadenomas, 3.8% were pseudocysts, and 2.5% were ductal adenocarcinomas.[19] Given that only 20.8% of the asymptomatic cysts in this series were completely benign, the fact that nonoperative management is controversial is understandable.[20] Nonetheless, ample literature supports surveillance of asymptomatic pancreatic cysts[21–28] as opposed to immediate surgical resection, because they grow extremely slowly, if at all, even if they are neoplastic.

The imaging-based decision whether to resect or observe a pancreatic cyst depends predominantly on cyst size. Most studies concur that the frequency of malignancy in a cyst smaller than 3 cm is extremely low, although some recommend 2.5 cm as a maximal diameter for nonsurgical management.[29] However, a significant percentage of these lesions smaller than 3 cm will be mucinous, but rarely is invasive cancer found in these lesions on resection.[25] Studies of patients in whom cysts have been resected or aspirated have found that malignancy or premalignancy does not correlate with cyst size alone; these studies consider mucinous lesions of any size to be premalignant.[18,20,30,31]

A retrospective case series reviewed 79 patients who underwent long-term follow-up, either for 5 years with imaging (n = 22) or 8 years with clinical follow-up (n = 27), who were diagnosed with small (≤2 cm) simple pancreatic cysts on sonography or CT from 1985 to 1996. Of the 22 patients who underwent radiologic follow-up, 13 (59%) had cysts that remained unchanged or became smaller

(mean size, 8 mm; mean follow-up, 9 years) and 9 (41%) had cysts that enlarged, from a mean of 14 mm to a mean of 26 mm (mean follow-up, 8 years). Of the 27 patients who underwent clinical or questionnaire follow-up (mean follow-up, 10 years), none developed symptomatic pancreatic disease. Eighteen patients (23%) died within 8 years without adequate radiologic follow-up, although none of pancreas-related causes.[32] This experience would support the surveillance of cysts smaller 3 cm regardless of origin.

Size alone cannot be an independent decision-making variable. Radiologists must attempt to exclude the presence of morphologic abnormalities that raise the specter of a complex cyst. Aside

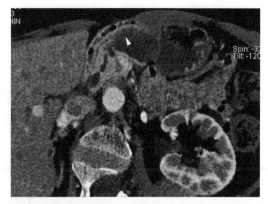

Fig. 3. Mural nodules. Ill-defined soft tissue density is seen along the superior aspect of this cyst (*arrowhead*). Mural nodules and irregularity may be difficult to appreciate on MDCT but may be more evident on MRI or endoscopic ultrasound. Because of these features combined with its size (4 cm in length), this lesion was considered surgical. Pathology showed only dysplasia, no carcinoma.

from a cyst larger than 3 cm, features that are worrisome include the presence of mural nodules, dilatation of the common bile duct, dilatation of the main pancreatic duct larger than 6 mm, duct wall enhancement, and lymphadenopathy[27,33–37] (Fig. 3).

When a cyst larger than 1 cm is detected, before a specific radiologic-based decision is made, a dedicated "pancreas-style" study should be performed. Because smaller cysts (closer to 1 cm) are more likely to be benign, the timing of this examination is better determined through clinical decision rather than according to a rigid algorithm. One could make a case for delaying the characterization study for several months[6–12] for lesions closer to 1 cm than to 3 cm. If MDCT is used for lesion characterization, a dual-phase acquisition in both pancreatic and portal venous phases using narrow detector configuration and intravenous contrast is the appropriate protocol. Thin-section images should be available on a workstation to facilitate three-dimensional analysis (Fig. 4). Alternatively, MRI performed at 1.5T can be used. The study should include sequences that display in and out of phase T1 and T2 (preferably with fat suppression), and fat suppressed three-dimensional gadolinium-enhanced sequences in pancreatic, portal, and equilibrium phases. Additionally, respiratory triggered three-dimensional MRCP is necessary.[38] Secretin administration may facilitate visualization of the cyst's communication with the main pancreatic duct.[39]

Many cysts are smaller than 10 mm. In a study of 421 cysts, 144 (34%) were in this size range.[40] Cysts of this size are frequently detected at MRI; they are not easily characterized through imaging.

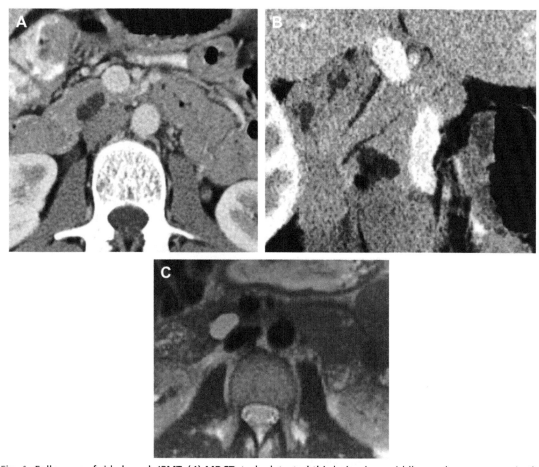

Fig. 4. Follow-up of side branch IPMT. (A) MDCT study detected this lesion in a middle-aged woman seen in the emergency department in 2003 for lower abdominal pain. (B) A "pancreatic-style" MDCT performed several weeks later study provided a data set that allowed creation of the CT pancreatogram confirming the diagnosis of IPMT. Because the lesion was smaller than 2 cm, the patient elected follow-up for the lesion. (C) The patient was advised to have the lesion followed up with MRI to decrease radiation exposure. This T2-weighted image was obtained in 2010; the lesion has not changed in the past 7 years.

Recommendations for following up these cysts cannot be made based on the appearance at imaging alone.

Non–imaging-based parameters are critical in the final recommendation to follow-up, resection, or ignore. The presence or absence of patient symptoms (eg, weight loss, jaundice, diabetes, anorexia) is a critical component of these decisions.[41] Lee and colleagues[42] found that in asymptomatic patients with pancreatic cysts smaller than 3 cm, the incidence of occult malignancy was 3.3%, whereas 90% of patients with malignant lesions were symptomatic.

The treatment philosophy of a given institution must also be factored into the decision-making process. A meta-analysis compared[1] initial pancreaticoduodenectomy,[2] yearly noninvasive radiographic surveillance,[3] yearly invasive surveillance with endoscopic ultrasound, and[4] the do-nothing approach for all cysts larger than 2 cm in the pancreatic head. Survival was maximized if all cysts were resected; however, when measuring quality-adjusted survival, the do-nothing approach maximized quality of life in patients younger than 75 years of age who had cysts smaller than 3 cm. Once age exceeded 85 years, noninvasive surveillance dominated. Initial pancreaticoduodenectomy did not maximize quality of life in any age group or cyst size.[43]

If the decision is made to resect a cyst smaller than 3 cm, every attempt should be made to determine a specific diagnosis. Endoscopic ultrasound with fine-needle aspiration is the most widely used technique to obtain cyst content for analysis. Cyst size is the primary determinate of successful aspiration.[44] A carcinoembryonic antigen level in the aspirate of 192 ng/mL has a high specificity for discriminating mucinous from nonmucinous

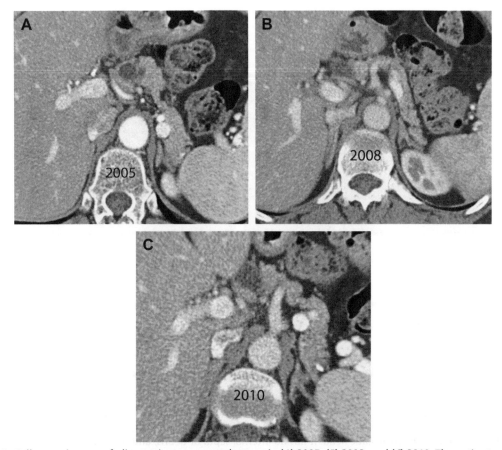

Fig. 5. Follow-up images of oligocystic serous cystadenoma in (A) 2005, (B) 2008, and (C) 2010. The patient was 56 years old in 2005. The lesion has been stable for the entire period of observation. Because of the size, the patient underwent an endoscopic ultrasound–assisted aspiration, which confirmed glycogen-rich serous fluid. The patient was dismissed from further follow-up this year; however, she was told that if she developed any pancreatic type symptoms, she would require reevaluation with further imaging.

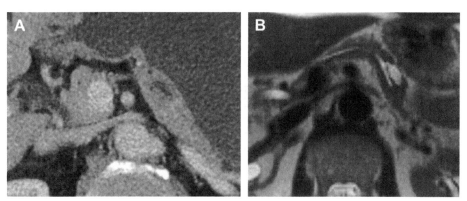

Fig. 6. (*A*) Irregular pancreatic body cyst is seen in this middle-aged man in 2006. No pancreas-related symptoms were present. The mass was somewhat irregular. Aspiration under endoscopic ultrasound was suggested; however, this procedure did not yield a diagnostic sample. Follow-up was advised. (*B*) Follow-up MRI in 2010. T2-weighted image clearly shows the mass to be a branch duct IPMT. The lesion has not increased in size in 4 years. Further follow-up is unnecessary if the patient remains asymptomatic.

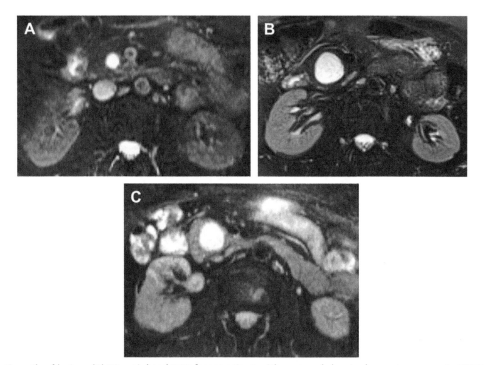

Fig. 7. Growth of lesion. (*A*) T2-weighted MRI from patient with vague abdominal symptoms seen in 2007 shows a high signal mass in the pancreatic head. It has no internal septa or debris, and the remainder of the pancreas was normal. Follow-up was recommended. (*B*) T2-weighted MRI in same patient from 2008. The mass has grown. An aspiration under endoscopic ultrasound guidance was attempted but was nondiagnostic. The patient elected to continue follow-up. (*C*) T2-weighted MRI in the same patient in 2009. Growth has continued. The lesion remains otherwise unchanged with no interval development of worrisome features. Surgery was recommended, and no new attempt at aspiration was made. The mass was a pseudocyst.

cysts, with an accuracy surpassing cyst morphology.[45,46] Amylase levels of less than 250 exclude pseudocyst. However, a high degree of overlap exists between the values obtained at aspiration.[47] There is variability among institutions in the ability to accurately analyze the often small volumes of pancreatic aspirate. The overall sensitivity of endoscopic ultrasound aspiration cytology is low; however, the specificity is adequate in differentiating mucinous from nonmucinous cystic lesions.[48]

WHAT IS THE BEST FOLLOW-UP METHOD?

Assuming that a lesion meets strictly applied criteria for follow-up (<3 cm, no mural nodules, no main pancreatic duct dilatation, asymptomatic), follow-up studies are often recommended in the radiologic report. Two questions are raised: what is the frequency of follow-up, and what is the optimal method of follow-up?

The frequency of follow-up examinations is not resolved. A conservative management would be to follow up a cyst for 24 months at 6-month intervals and then yearly for a second 24 months, declaring stability after 4 years.[49] The Sendai guidelines recommend all cysts smaller than 1 cm be followed each year, all cysts from 1 to 2 cm followed as described earlier, cysts from 2 to 3 cm be followed every 3 to 6 months, and all cysts larger than 3 cm be resected.[23] Based on longitudinal observation of 166 cysts in 150 patients, a second approach suggests having the first follow-up occur 2 years after baseline.[40] American College of Radiology (ACR) guidelines recommend a single follow-up in 1 year for lesions smaller than 2 cm; a follow-up of every 6 months for 2 years and then yearly for lesions 2 to 3 cm; and for lesions larger than 3 cm, resect unless they are serous cystadenoma or proven to be pseudocyst through aspiration. All of these guidelines suggest that patients must remain asymptomatic during the follow-up period (Fig. 5).

The choice of follow-up method is important. The ACR subcommittee on incidental pancreatic lesions recommends MRI as the preferred follow-up procedure based on superior contrast resolution making the detection of septa, nodules, and main pancreatic duct communication easiest to recognize[17] and the lack of ionizing radiation[50] (Fig. 6). Cost and resource availability must be factored into this decision. For patients older than 60 years, radiation issues may not be as compelling. Regardless of the choice of follow-up procedure, care must be taken to assure that measurements are made carefully and consistently.[51] The lesion must be carefully measured;

not only must the slice number and series appear in the report but also electronic calipers must be placed on the exact image used to determine the diameters. Currently, no consensus has defined growth. The precision of manual measurement is well-known to be inversely related to the lesion diameter. Thus, determining whether the reported growth of a small lesion is true growth or measurement error may be difficult. Considerable research is currently evaluating semiautomated lesion segmentation, which will overcome this problem.[52] Growth alone may not be sufficient to recommend surgery; the authors believe that cyst content should be aspirated before surgical excision is performed (Fig. 7).

Recent reports have documented ductal adenocarcinoma developing in a remote site within the pancreas from a known branch duct IPMT.[53,54] This finding is not surprising in that many believe the presence of a mucinous lesion is a signal of increased risk of pancreatic neoplasm anywhere within the gland. In most of these cases, the target cyst remains unchanged. The development of these lesions is thought to reflect a field effect within the pancreas, with the cyst being a signal of a gland that is at risk for developing carcinoma. Increased numbers of pancreatic intraepithelial neoplasia lesions, believed to be precursor lesions for development of ductal adenocarcinoma, are

---

Box 1
Recommendations for radiologists confronted with an incidental pancreatic cyst

1. Surgery should be considered for patients with cysts larger than 3 cm.
2. If the lesion is a serous cystadenoma, surgery is deferred until the cyst is larger than 4 cm.
3. Patients with simple cysts smaller than 3 cm can be followed up, but attempts should be made to characterize cysts larger than 2 cm at detection; if this cannot be done based on the available imaging study, MRI is the preferred procedure.
4. Cysts smaller than 1 cm cannot be further characterized by imaging, but can be followed up less frequently than cysts larger than 3 cm; in elderly patients (>80 years of age), these cysts likely will not require further investigation.
5. Aspiration is strongly advised to exclude pseudocyst before any surgery is performed.
6. Patients must remain asymptomatic during the follow-up period.

From Berland LL, Silverman SG, Gore RM, et al. Managing incidental findings on abdominal CT: white paper of the ACR incidental findings committee. J Am Coll Radiol 2010;7(10):754–73.

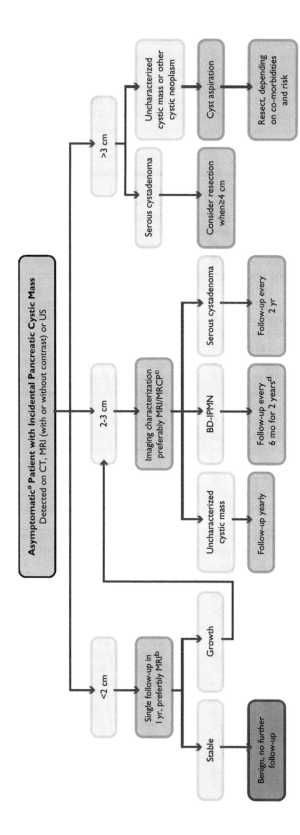

Fig. 8. Flow chart for imaging workup of incidental pancreatic masses in asymptomatic patients. As with all guidelines, these are not meant to be a rigid set of rules, but rather a starting point for clinically relevant decision making. BD-IPMN, branch duct intraductal papillary mucinous neoplasm; US, ultrasound. [a] Signs and symptoms include hyperamylasemia, recent onset diabetes, severe epigastric pain, weight loss, steatorrhea, or jaundice. [b] Consider decreasing interval if younger, omitting with limited life expectancy. Recommend limited T2-weighted MRI for routine follow-ups. [c] Recommend pancreas-dedicated MRI with MRCP. [d] If no growth after 2 years, follow yearly. If growth or suspicious features develop, consider resection. (From Berland LL, Silverman SG, Gore RM, et al. Managing incidental findings on abdominal CT: white paper of the ACR incidental findings committee. J Am Coll Radiol 2010;7(10):754–73.)

seen in resected specimens.[55] Should a significant frequency of cancer develop elsewhere in the pancreas of patients with any type of cyst, follow-up imaging recommendations and surgical management of the cysts will be altered.

RECOMMENDATIONS FOR RADIOLOGISTS

The pancreas subcommittee of the ACR committee on incidental lesions developed the following recommendations for radiologists confronted with an incidental pancreatic cyst (a cyst seen in an asymptomatic patient (Box 1).

These are recommendations, not guidelines nor care standards. Fig. 8 provides these recommendations in flow-chart format. Individual patient characteristics must be factored into every decision. Many clinicians who read this probably know of single case examples that are contrary to the above recommendations. However, the extensive observational experience of the authors and concordant experience documented in the published literature validate the approach outlined in this article as a reasonable departure point for analyzing patients with incidental pancreatic cysts.

REFERENCES

1. Spinelli KS, Fromwiller TE, Daniel RA, et al. Cystic pancreatic neoplasms: observe or operate. Ann Surg 2004;239(5):651–7 [discussion: 657–9].
2. Laffan TA, Horton KM, Klein AP, et al. Prevalence of unsuspected pancreatic cysts on MDCT. AJR Am J Roentgenol 2008;191(3):802–7.
3. Zhang XM, Mitchell DG, Dohke M, et al. Pancreatic cysts: depiction on single-shot fast spin-echo MR images. Radiology 2002;223(2):547–53.
4. Lee KS, Sekhar A, Rofsky NM, et al. Prevalence of incidental pancreatic cysts in the adult population on MR imaging. Am J Gastroenterol 2010;2010:30.
5. Simeone DM. SSAT/AGA/ASGE state of the art conference on cystic neoplasms of the pancreas. J Gastrointest Surg 2008;12(8):1475–7.
6. Adsay NV. Cystic neoplasia of the pancreas: pathology and biology. J Gastrointest Surg 2008; 12(3):401–4.
7. Parra-Herran CE, Garcia MT, Herrera L, et al. Cystic lesions of the pancreas: clinical and pathologic review of cases in a five year period. JOP 2010; 11(4):358–64.
8. Procacci C, Graziani R, Bicego E, et al. Serous cystadenoma of the pancreas: report of 30 cases with emphasis on the imaging findings. J Comput Assist Tomogr 1997;21(3):373–82.
9. Procacci C, Biasiutti C, Carbognin G, et al. Characterization of cystic tumors of the pancreas: CT accuracy. J Comput Assist Tomogr 1999;23(6):906–12.
10. Rautou PE, Levy P, Vullierme MP, et al. Morphologic changes in branch duct intraductal papillary mucinous neoplasms of the pancreas: a midterm follow-up study. Clin Gastroenterol Hepatol 2008; 6(7):807–14.
11. Procacci C, Carbognin G, Accordini S, et al. CT features of malignant mucinous cystic tumors of the pancreas. Eur Radiol 2001;11(9):1626–30.
12. Choi JY, Kim MJ, Lee JY, et al. Typical and atypical manifestations of serous cystadenoma of the pancreas: imaging findings with pathologic correlation. AJR Am J Roentgenol 2009;193(1):136–42.
13. Cohen-Scali F, Vilgrain V, Brancatelli G, et al. Discrimination of unilocular macrocystic serous cystadenoma from pancreatic pseudocyst and mucinous cystadenoma with CT: initial observations. Radiology 2003;228(3):727–33.
14. Sahani DV, Kadavigere R, Saokar A, et al. Cystic pancreatic lesions: a simple imaging-based classification system for guiding management. Radiographics 2005;25(6):1471–84.
15. Walsh RM, Henderson JM, Vogt DP, et al. Prospective preoperative determination of mucinous pancreatic cystic neoplasms. Surgery 2002;132(4):628–33 [discussion: 633–4].
16. Takeshita K, Kutomi K, Takada K, et al. Unusual imaging appearances of pancreatic serous cystadenoma: correlation with surgery and pathologic analysis. Abdom Imaging 2005;15:15.
17. Waters JA, Schmidt CM, Pinchot JW, et al. CT vs MRCP: optimal classification of IPMN type and extent. J Gastrointest Surg 2008;12(1):101–9.
18. Correa-Gallego C, Ferrone CR, Thayer SP, et al. Incidental pancreatic cysts: do we really know what we are watching? Pancreatology 2010; 10(2–3):144–50.
19. Fernandez-del Castillo C, Targarona J, Thayer SP, et al. Incidental pancreatic cysts: clinicopathologic characteristics and comparison with symptomatic patients. Arch Surg 2003;138(4):427–33 [discussion: 433–4].
20. Walsh RM, Vogt DP, Henderson JM, et al. Management of suspected pancreatic cystic neoplasms based on cyst size. Surgery 2008;144(4):677–84 [discussion: 684–5].
21. Lahav M, Maor Y, Avidan B, et al. Nonsurgical management of asymptomatic incidental pancreatic cysts. Clin Gastroenterol Hepatol 2007;5(7):813–7.
22. Sahani DV, Saokar A, Hahn PF, et al. Pancreatic cysts 3 cm or smaller: how aggressive should treatment be? Radiology 2006;238(3):912–9.
23. Tanaka M, Chari S, Adsay V, et al. International consensus guidelines for management of intraductal papillary mucinous neoplasms and mucinous cystic

neoplasms of the pancreas. Pancreatology 2006; 6(1–2):17–32.

24. Walsh RM, Vogt DP, Henderson JM, et al. Natural history of indeterminate pancreatic cysts. Surgery 2005;138(4):665–70 [discussion: 670–1].

25. Allen PJ, D'Angelica M, Gonen M, et al. A selective approach to the resection of cystic lesions of the pancreas: results from 539 consecutive patients. Ann Surg 2006;244(4):572–82.

26. Edirimanne S, Connor SJ. Incidental pancreatic cystic lesions. World J Surg 2008;32(9):2028–37.

27. Brounts LR, Lehmann RK, Causey MW, et al. Natural course and outcome of cystic lesions in the pancreas. Am J Surg 2009;197(5):619–22 [discussion: 622–3].

28. Bassi C, Sarr MG, Lillemoe KD, et al. Natural history of intraductal papillary mucinous neoplasms (IPMN): current evidence and implications for management. J Gastrointest Surg 2008;12(4):645–50.

29. Gomez D, Rahman SH, Wong LF, et al. Predictors of malignant potential of cystic lesions of the pancreas. Eur J Surg Oncol 2008;34(8):876–82.

30. Ceppa EP, De la Fuente SG, Reddy SK, et al. Defining criteria for selective operative management of pancreatic cystic lesions: does size really matter? J Gastrointest Surg 2010;14(2):236–44.

31. Goh BK, Tan YM, Cheow PC, et al. Cystic lesions of the pancreas: an appraisal of an aggressive resectional policy adopted at a single institution during 15 years. Am J Surg 2006;192(2):148–54.

32. Handrich SJ, Hough DM, Fletcher JG, et al. The natural history of the incidentally discovered small simple pancreatic cyst: long-term follow-up and clinical implications. AJR Am J Roentgenol 2005;184(1):20–3.

33. Lee SH, Shin CM, Park JK, et al. Outcomes of cystic lesions in the pancreas after extended follow-up. Dig Dis Sci 2007;52(10):2653–9.

34. Salvia R, Crippa S, Falconi M, et al. Branch-duct intraductal papillary mucinous neoplasms of the pancreas: to operate or not to operate? Gut 2007; 56(8):1086–90.

35. Bassi C, Crippa S, Salvia R. Intraductal papillary mucinous neoplasms (IPMNs): is it time to (sometimes) spare the knife? Gut 2008;57(3):287–9.

36. Javle M, Shah P, Yu J, et al. Cystic pancreatic tumors (CPT): predictors of malignant behavior. J Surg Oncol 2007;95(3):221–8.

37. Manfredi R, Graziani R, Motton M, et al. Main pancreatic duct intraductal papillary mucinous neoplasms: accuracy of MR imaging in differentiation between benign and malignant tumors compared with histopathologic analysis. Radiology 2009;253(1):106–15.

38. Sodickson A, Mortele KJ, Barish MA, et al. Three-dimensional fast-recovery fast spin-echo MRCP: comparison with two-dimensional single-shot fast spin-echo techniques. Radiology 2006;238(2):549–59.

39. Carbognin G, Pinali L, Girardi V, et al. Collateral branches IPMTs: secretin-enhanced MRCP. Abdom Imaging 2007;32(3):374–80.

40. Das A, Wells CD, Nguyen CC. Incidental cystic neoplasms of pancreas: what is the optimal interval of imaging surveillance? Am J Gastroenterol 2008; 103(7):1657–62.

41. Taouli B, Vilgrain V, Vullierme MP, et al. Intraductal papillary mucinous tumors of the pancreas: helical CT with histopathologic correlation. Radiology 2000;217(3):757–64.

42. Lee CJ, Scheiman J, Anderson MA, et al. Risk of malignancy in resected cystic tumors of the pancreas < or =3 cm in size: is it safe to observe asymptomatic patients? A multi-institutional report. J Gastrointest Surg 2008;12(2):234–42.

43. Weinberg BM, Spiegel BM, Tomlinson JS, et al. Asymptomatic pancreatic cystic neoplasms: maximizing survival and quality of life using Markov-based clinical nomograms. Gastroenterology 2010; 138(2):531–40.

44. Walsh RM, Zuccaro G, Dumot JA, et al. Predicting success of endoscopic aspiration for suspected pancreatic cystic neoplasms. JOP 2008;9(5):612–7.

45. Brugge WR, Lewandrowski K, Lee-Lewandrowski E, et al. Diagnosis of pancreatic cystic neoplasms: a report of the cooperative pancreatic cyst study. Gastroenterology 2004;126(5):1330–6.

46. Linder JD, Geenen JE, Catalano MF. Cyst fluid analysis obtained by EUS-guided FNA in the evaluation of discrete cystic neoplasms of the pancreas: a prospective single-center experience. Gastrointest Endosc 2006;64(5):697–702.

47. van der Waaij LA, van Dullemen HM, Porte RJ. Cyst fluid analysis in the differential diagnosis of pancreatic cystic lesions: a pooled analysis. Gastrointest Endosc 2005;62(3):383–9.

48. Thosani N, Thosani S, Qiao W, et al. Role of EUS-FNA-based cytology in the diagnosis of mucinous pancreatic cystic lesions: a systematic review and meta-analysis. Dig Dis Sci 2010;55(10):2756–66.

49. Salvia R, Crippa S, Partelli S, et al. Pancreatic cystic tumours: when to resect, when to observe. Eur Rev Med Pharmacol Sci 2010;14(4):395–406.

50. Macari M, Lee T, Kim S, et al. Is gadolinium necessary for MRI follow-up evaluation of cystic lesions in the pancreas? Preliminary results. AJR Am J Roentgenol 2009;192(1):159–64.

51. Maimone S, Agrawal D, Pollack MJ, et al. Variability in measurements of pancreatic cyst size among EUS, CT, and magnetic resonance imaging modalities. Gastrointest Endosc 2010;71(6):945–50.

52. Pauls S, Kurschner C, Dharaiya E, et al. Comparison of manual and automated size measurements of lung metastases on MDCT images: potential influence on therapeutic decisions. Eur J Radiol 2008; 66(1):19–26.

53. Tada M, Kawabe T, Arizumi M, et al. Pancreatic cancer in patients with pancreatic cystic lesions: a prospective study in 197 patients. Clin Gastroenterol Hepatol 2006;4(10):1265–70.

54. Uehara H, Nakaizumi A, Ishikawa O, et al. Development of ductal carcinoma of the pancreas during follow-up of branch duct intraductal papillary mucinous neoplasm of the pancreas. Gut 2008; 57(11):1561–5.

55. Takaori K, Kobashi Y, Matsusue S, et al. Clinico-pathological features of pancreatic intraepithelial neoplasias and their relationship to intraductal papillary-mucinous tumors. J Hepatobiliary Pancreat Surg 2003;10(2):125–36.

Incidentally Discovered Adrenal Mass

Julie H. Song, MD*, William W. Mayo-Smith, MD

KEYWORDS

• Adrenal • Adrenal incidentaloma • Adrenal mass

As use of cross-sectional imaging continues to rise, adrenal masses are frequently detected incidentally in the daily practice of radiology. These adrenal masses, commonly referred to as *adrenal incidentalomas*, are asymptomatic masses ($\geq$1 cm) discovered on imaging studies performed for reasons unrelated to adrenal disease. The prevalence of incidental adrenal mass at CT is approximately 4% to 5%,[1–3] reflecting the estimated prevalence in the general population of 3% to 7%.[4–6] Most of these incidentally found masses are benign, with adenomas the most common pathology.[7–9] However, the adrenal gland is a common site of metastasis, and also of clinical concern are primary adrenal neoplasms that require intervention, such as pheochromocytoma, aldosteronomas, cortisol-producing adenoma, and adrenal cortical carcinoma. Once an adrenal mass is detected, the goal of adrenal imaging is to characterize and differentiate the benign "leave-alone" lesions from masses that require treatment without exhaustive workup. This article discusses contemporary adrenal imaging and the optimal algorithm for the workup of incidentally discovered adrenal masses. The recommendations presented were recently published in the *Journal of the American College of Radiology*,[10] and readers are also directed to a recent comprehensive review on this topic.[11]

CLINICAL IMPLICATION: BENIGN VERSUS MALIGNANT

When an adrenal mass is discovered incidentally, the main diagnostic dilemma is whether it is malignant. Several factors pertaining to the risk of malignancy determine the imaging workup, including imaging features, lesion size, change in size, and the clinical context in which the adrenal lesion is discovered, particularly with regard to patient history of malignancy. Certain imaging features are suspicious for malignancy, such as central necrosis, heterogeneous attenuation, and irregular margins. In general, benign adrenal masses are of homogenous low density with smooth margins. Certain adrenal lesions have specific benign imaging features that are diagnostic at detection and do not warrant further workup. Adrenal myelolipomas are easily recognized by the presence of macroscopic fat (Fig. 1), and adrenal cysts can be diagnosed when a mass appears as a simple cyst without enhancement. Prior studies are extremely helpful, because stability implies benignity, and therefore every effort should be made to compare with prior studies before recommending additional imaging workup. In general, an enlarging adrenal mass is considered malignant. Although no specific size criterion reliably distinguishes a benign from a malignant mass, the risk of malignancy increases with the size of the mass. In patients without history of malignancy, the main concern for a large adrenal mass is adrenal cortical carcinoma, although it is rare in the general population, with estimated prevalence of 0.6 to 2 per million.[7] Typically, adrenal masses larger than 4 cm are surgically resected in patients without history of malignancy, unless a definitive benign diagnosis, such as myelolipoma, adrenal cyst, typical adenoma, or hemorrhage, can be established.[9]

Department of Diagnostic Imaging, Rhode Island Hospital—Warren Alpert Medical School of Brown University, 593 Eddy Street, Providence, RI 02903, USA
* Corresponding author.
E-mail address: jsong2@lifespan.org

Radiol Clin N Am 49 (2011) 361–368
doi:10.1016/j.rcl.2010.10.006

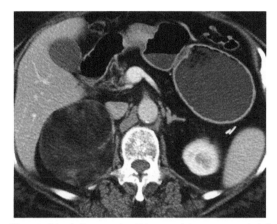

Fig. 1. Myelolipoma in 74-year-old woman. Axial contrast-enhanced CT image shows a 9-cm right adrenal mass containing a large amount of fat and a small component of soft tissue, diagnostic of a myelolipoma.

Patient history of malignancy is one of the most important determinants in the workup of incidental adrenal lesion. It is extremely rare for an incidental adrenal mass to be metastatic disease of unrecognized primary malignancy.[12,13] In one study of 1049 incidental adrenal masses in patients with no history of cancer, there were no malignant lesions.[3] However, in oncologic patients, the rate of metastatic disease depends on the type of primary malignancy. In these patients, workup of an incidental adrenal mass depends on overall patient status. In patients with evidence of widespread metastatic disease, the workup of an adrenal mass is of unlikely benefit. However, differentiating a benign from metastatic adrenal mass in patients in whom the adrenal gland is the only potential site of metastasis would be important, because the diagnosis may alter prognosis and treatment options. For example, in a patient with a potentially resectable lung carcinoma and an isolated adrenal mass, differentiating a benign adenoma from a metastasis is critical for accurate staging to determine optimal treatment (curative resection vs chemotherapy, respectively). The overall clinical context in which the adrenal mass is detected is also important to consider. In a patient with a limited life expectancy or severe comorbidities, the workup of an incidental adrenal mass may not be appropriate.

IMAGING EVALUATION: CT, MRI, AND POSITRON EMISSION TOMOGRAPHY

CT and MRI are the most commonly used imaging studies for evaluating an incidental adrenal mass, with positron emission tomography (PET) usually

reserved for patients with known extra-adrenal malignancy. These images reflect physiologic differences distinguishing adenoma from malignant masses, such as intracytoplasmic lipid content, contrast washout pattern, and metabolic activity.

Lee and colleagues[14] reported the first large series distinguishing benign from malignant adrenal masses based on density measurement on unenhanced CT. Adrenal adenomas have a varying amount of intracytoplasmic lipid, and an inverse relationship exists between the lipid content of the adenoma and its density measurement on CT.[15] Approximately 70% of adenomas have sufficient intracytoplasmic lipid to be diagnosed on unenhanced CT. A meta-analysis showed that a threshold of 10 HU allowed adenoma to be diagnosed with 71% sensitivity and 98% specificity, and therefore this is currently the standard threshold used to diagnose a lipid-rich adenoma on CT (**Fig. 2**).[16]

More recently, the same principle of intracytoplasmic lipid was used in histogram analysis to diagnose adenoma on unenhanced and contrast-enhanced CT. Using this method, the percentage of negative pixels within the region of interest is measured. Bae and colleagues[17] achieved increased sensitivity in diagnosing adenoma compared with the 10-HU threshold method, while maintaining specificity at 100%. However, this method is not routinely used in clinical practice because of differing results on follow-up studies.[9,11]

Other CT parameters used to differentiate adenoma from nonadenoma are based on their different contrast washout characteristics.[18,19] After enhancement with intravenous contrast, adenomas lose contrast more rapidly while the

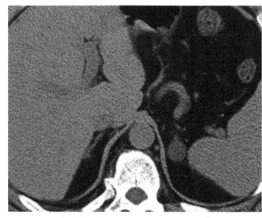

Fig. 2. Lipid-rich adenoma in 47-year-old man. Axial unenhanced CT image shows a well-defined 1.8-cm left adrenal mass with attenuation of 2 HU.

washout of metastasis is more prolonged. Korobkin and colleagues[18] showed that through calculating the percentage washout of initial enhancement and choosing an optimal threshold at 15 minutes, adenoma can be distinguished from nonadenomas. The accuracy of washout analysis has since been corroborated on multiple subsequent studies, although time chosen for delay scan was variable.[20-23] Absolute percentage washout (APW) values are calculated as follows and a value of 60% or greater at 15 minutes is diagnostic of an adenoma (Fig. 3):

$$APW = \frac{(enhanced\ HU) - (15\ min\ delayed\ HU)}{(enhanced\ HU) - (unenhanced\ HU)} \times 100\%$$

In the absence of unenhanced series, a relative percentage washout (RPW) can be calculated by the formula:

$$RPW = \frac{(enhanced\ HU) - (15\ min\ delayed\ HU)}{(enhanced\ HU)} \times 100\%$$

An RPW value greater than 40% is diagnostic of adenoma.[18,21] Contrast washout is independent of the amount of lipid content and allows accurate diagnosis of both lipid-rich and lipid-poor adenoma.[20,23]

The principle MR technique used in adrenal evaluation is chemical shift imaging obtained as dual-echo breath-hold gradient echo acquisition. Similar to CT density measurement, this technique depends on the presence of intracytoplasmic lipid in adenomas to separate them from nonadenomas.[24,25] Chemical shift MRI (CS-MR) exploits the different resonant frequency rates of protons in fat and water molecules, with fat protons resonating at a slower frequency. By choosing the "correct" TE (echo time), the signal from lipid will oppose that from water, causing signal drop-off in voxels containing both lipid and water on opposed-phase imaging. Most adrenal adenomas containing sufficient amount of lipid lose signal (become darker) on the opposed-phase images compared with the spleen (Fig. 4). With CS-MR, adenomas are differentiated from metastasis with sensitivity and specificity of 81%

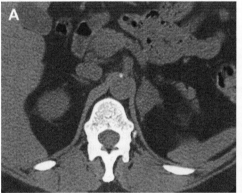
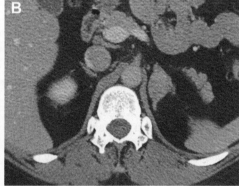
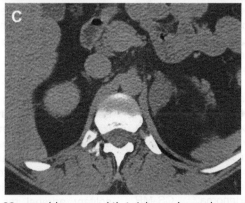

Fig. 3. Lipid-poor adenoma in 38-year-old woman. (A) Axial unenhanced scan shows 2.6-cm left adrenal mass with attenuation of 22 HU. (B) On dynamic contrast-enhanced phase scan, adrenal mass enhances to 90 HU. (C) On 15-minute delayed scan, adrenal mass attenuation is 37 HU. Absolute percent washout and relative percent washout are 78% and 59%, respectively, diagnostic of an adenoma.

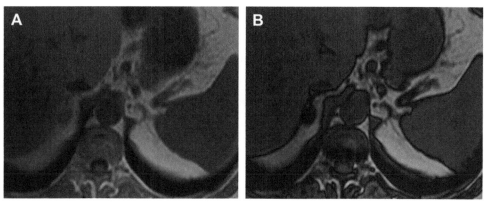

Fig. 4. 1.5-cm right adrenal adenoma in 67-year-old man. (*A*) T1-weighted in-phase MR image shows a right adrenal mass that is mildly hyperintense relative to the spleen. (*B*) T1-weighted opposed-phase MR image shows marked signal intensity loss relative to the spleen, diagnostic of an adenoma. Note the presence of mild hepatic steatosis.

to 100% and 94% to 100%, respectively.[11,26] The paired in-phase and opposed-phase images can be analyzed using quantitative methods such as signal intensity index or chemical shift ratio.[27,28] However, because simple visual analysis is as effective and easier to use, it is more commonly used in clinical practice.[29] Occasionally, heterogeneous signal suppression may be seen in an adenoma because of a heterogeneous population of lipid-rich cells.[30]

In a few studies comparing unenhanced CT with CS-MR, CS-MR allowed additional diagnosis of adenoma that was lipid-poor on CT.[31,32] Israel and colleagues[31] reported that 62% of adenomas with greater than 10 HU were characterized as adenoma, and Haider and colleagues[32] reported that 89% of adenoma with CT density measurement between 10 and 30 HU were correctly diagnosed using CS-MR. However, when comparing methods of washout characteristics with lipid content of adenoma, Park and colleagues[33] showed that delayed enhanced CT was superior to CS-MR in a small series. Although the rapid contrast washout characteristics of adenoma were first described with gadolinium-enhanced MR with promising results,[34] subsequent studies have not validated these findings for clinical use.[35]

Currently, adrenal CT with combined unenhanced and delayed enhanced CT seems to be the most powerful and widely used single imaging tool in the workup of adrenal masses.[11,21,22] In one study of 166 adrenal masses, the combined adrenal protocol was 96% accurate in distinguishing adenoma from nonadenoma.[21] CS-MR remains a useful tool in patients in whom iodinated contrast is contraindicated because of allergy or renal insufficiency or in young patients in whom

radiation exposure is a concern, because most adrenal adenomas are lipid-rich and will be diagnosed with CS-MR.

PET and PET-CT using fluorine-18-2fluoro-2-deoxy-D-glucose (FDG) is becoming a standard staging evaluation to identify metastasis in many oncologic patients. In general, metastases has increased FDG uptake because of increased glucose use, and most adrenal metastases show increased activity relative to the liver (Fig. 5), whereas most benign adenomas do not. PET-CT further improves diagnostic performance through incorporating CT density measurement analysis of an adrenal mass and allowing its accurate localization. PET and PET-CT can be used to differentiate benign from malignant adrenal masses in patients with cancer, with a sensitivity and specificity ranging from 93% to 100% and 90% to 100%, respectively.[36–39] Because a small number of adrenal adenomas and other benign lesions can show slightly increased uptake, more recent studies suggest the specificity is closer to 95%.[11,38]

ADRENAL BIOPSY

The number of imaging-guided biopsies necessary to diagnose an adrenal mass has decreased because of recent advances in imaging characterization of an adrenal mass.[40] However, biopsy may still be necessary to exclude metastasis if imaging findings are inconclusive, or to evaluate enlarging adrenal masses. Adrenal biopsy can also be used to confirm metastasis in patients with suspected solitary adrenal metastasis. Adrenal biopsy is usually performed with CT guidance and has been shown to be safe, with a 85% to 96% diagnostic accuracy and 3% to 9% complication

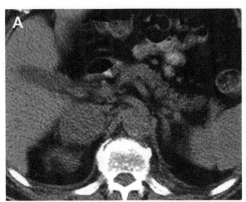
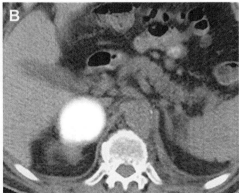

Fig. 5. Adrenal metastasis in 82-year-old man with non-small cell lung cancer. (A) Axial unenhanced CT image shows a 5-cm right adrenal mass. (B) Axial CT and PET coregistered image shows markedly increased FDG uptake in the right adrenal metastasis.

rate.[40–42] Before biopsy, the plasma-free metanephrine level should be obtained if the possibility exists that the adrenal mass is a pheochromocytoma. Biopsy of pheochromocytoma is generally avoided because it may induce hypertensive crisis.

DIAGNOSTIC ALGORITHM OF AN INCIDENTAL ADRENAL MASS (≥1 CM)

A recent adrenal imaging algorithm from the White Paper of the American College of Radiology (ACR) Committee on Incidental Findings is presented in Fig. 6.[10] This guideline also follows the recommendation of ACR Appropriateness Criteria.[9] If an incidental adrenal mass of any size has diagnostic features of a benign lesion, such as a myelolipoma, cyst, or a lipid-rich adenoma, a specific benign diagnosis can be made and no additional imaging is needed. Adrenal masses smaller than 4 cm with nondiagnostic imaging features for which prior imaging is available and that have been stable for at least a year are likely benign and do not need follow-up imaging. However, if the lesion is enlarging, biopsy or resection should be considered because the mass may be malignant.

In patients with no history of cancer, if no prior CT or MRI is available for comparison and the lesion has benign imaging features (low density, homogeneous with smooth margins), then the mass can be presumed to be benign and a follow-up unenhanced CT or CS-MR in 12 months may be considered. However, if suspicious imaging features are present, unenhanced CT or CS-MR could be performed. If these are not diagnostic of an adenoma, then adrenal CT protocol with washout analysis may be helpful. If the lesion does not have imaging and washout features of a benign lesion, then biopsy may be appropriate.

In oncology patients, if the adrenal mass does not have imaging features diagnostic of a benign lesion and no prior imaging is available to establish stability, unenhanced CT, CS-MR, or PET/PET-CT can be considered. If these studies do not confirm the mass to be an adenoma, then adrenal CT with washout analysis may be helpful. If these imaging studies are not diagnostic of a benign lesion, then biopsy should be considered.

An adrenal mass larger than 4 cm without a definitive benign diagnosis is usually resected in patients without history of cancer, because there is concern for an adrenal cortical carcinoma. In patients with a history of cancer, PET/PET-CT or biopsy is recommended because the large adrenal mass could represent a metastasis.

ENDOCRINOLOGIC FUNCTION

Imaging studies are useful in separating benign from malignant masses, but they do not address the functional status of an adrenal incidentaloma. Subclinical hyperfunction by an incidental adrenal mass is a recognized phenomenon, and some endocrinologists recommend excluding occult, asymptomatic, hyperfunctioning neoplasms in all adrenal incidentalomas through biochemical assays in addition to complete history and physical examination.[4–6] However, biochemical workup is costly and not routinely performed by many physicians because functioning tumors are uncommon among incidentalomas. If the imaging findings are consistent with an adenoma, biochemical assays may be appropriate if clinical signs and symptoms indicate adrenal hyperfunction.

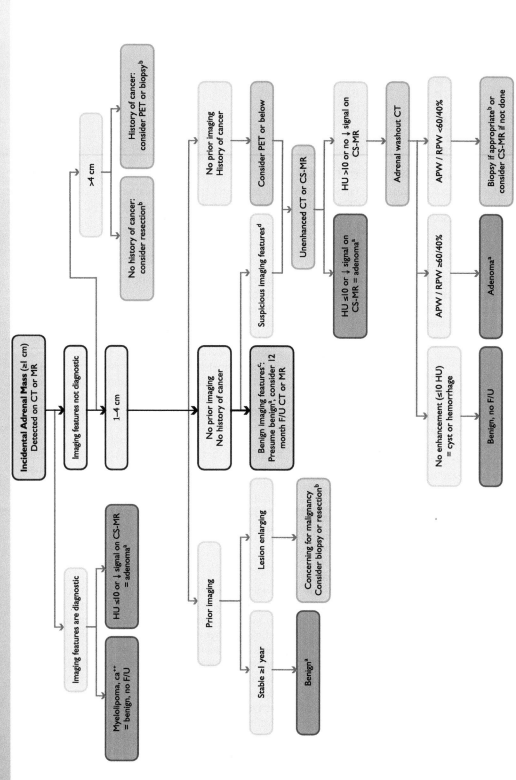

Fig. 6. Recommended algorithm for management of incidental adrenal masses as proposed by American College of Radiology. ↓, decreased; APW, absolute percentage washout; CS-MR, chemical shift MRI; F/U, follow-up. HU, Hounsfield unit; RPW, relative percentage washout; [a] If patient has clinical signs or symptoms of adrenal hyperfunction, consider biochemical evaluation. [b] Consider biochemical testing to exclude pheochromocytoma. [c] Benign imaging features: homogeneous, low density, smooth margins. [d] Suspicious imaging features: heterogeneous, necrosis, irregular margins. (*From* Berland LL, Silverman SG, Gore RM, et al. Managing incidental findings on abdominal CT: White Paper of the American College of Radiology Incidental Findings Committee. *J Am Coll Radiol* 2010;7(10):756–73; with permission.)

SUMMARY

Adrenal incidentalomas are common findings in contemporary cross-sectional imaging, and most are benign. Several imaging studies are in the armamentarium that could be used to accurately diagnose these masses. Judicious use of these studies will allow appropriate management of these common lesions.

REFERENCES

1. Kloos RT, Gross MD, Francis IR, et al. Incidentally discovered adrenal masses. Endocr Rev 1995;16: 460–84.
2. Bovio S, Cataldi A, Reimondo G, et al. Prevalence of adrenal incidentaloma in a contemporary computerized tomography series. J Endocrinol Invest 2006; 29:298–302.
3. Song JH, Chaudhry FS, Mayo-Smith WW. The incidental adrenal mass on CT: prevalence of adrenal disease in 1,049 consecutive adrenal masses in patients with no known malignancy. AJR Am J Roentgenol 2008;190:1163–8.
4. NIH state-of-the-science statement on management of the clinically inapparent adrenal mass ("incidentaloma"). NIH Consens State Sci Statements 2002;19: 1–25.
5. Grumbach MM, Biller BM, Braunstein GD, et al. Management of the clinically inapparent adrenal mass ("incidentaloma"). NIH conference. Ann Intern Med 2003;138:424–9.
6. Young WF Jr. The incidentally discovered adrenal mass. N Engl J Med 2007;356:601–10.
7. Mansmann G, Lau J, Balk E, et al. The clinically inapparent adrenal mass: update in diagnosis and management. Endocr Rev 2004;25:309–40.
8. Barzon L, Sonino N, Fallo F, et al. Prevalence and natural history of adrenal incidentalomas. Eur J Endocrinol 2003;149:273–85.
9. Francis IR, Casalino DD, Arellano RS, et al. Incidentally discovered adrenal mass. American College of Radiology. ACR appropriateness criteria 2009. Available at: http://www.acr.org/SecondaryMainMe nuCategories/quality_safety/app_criteria/pdf/ExpertP anelonUrologicImaging/IncidentallyDiscoveredAdren alMassDoc7.aspx. Accessed October 30, 2010.
10. Berland LL, Silverman SG, Gore RM, et al. Managing incidental findings on abdominal CT: White Paper of the American College of Radiology Incidental Findings Committee. J Am Coll Radiol 2010;7(10):754–73.
11. Boland GW, Blake MA, Hahn PF, et al. Incidental adrenal lesions: principles, techniques, and algorithms for imaging characterization. Radiology 2008;249:756–75.
12. Herrera MF, Grant CS, van Heerden JA, et al. Incidentally discovered adrenal tumors: an institutional perspective. Surgery 1991;110:1014–21.
13. Lee JE, Evans DB, Hickey RC, et al. Unknown primary cancer presenting as an adrenal mass: frequency and implications for diagnostic evaluation of adrenal incidentalomas. Surgery 1998;124:1115–22.
14. Lee MJ, Hahn PF, Papanicolaou N, et al. Benign and malignant adrenal masses: CT distinction with attenuation coefficients, size and observer analysis. Radiology 1991;179:415–8.
15. Korobkin M, Giordano TJ, Brodeur FJ, et al. Adrenal adenomas: relationship between histologic lipid and CT and MR findings. Radiology 1996;200:743–7.
16. Boland GW, Lee MJ, Gazelle GS, et al. Characterization of adrenal masses using unenhanced CT: an analysis of the CT literature. AJR Am J Roentgenol 1998;171:201–4.
17. Bae KT, Fuangtharnthip P, Prasad SR, et al. Adrenal masses: CT characterization with histogram analysis method. Radiology 2003;228:735–42.
18. Korobkin M, Brodeur FJ, Francis IR, et al. CT time-attenuation washout curves of adrenal adenomas and nonadenomas. AJR Am J Roentgenol 1998; 170:747–52.
19. Szolar DH, Kammerhuber FH. Adrenal adenomas and nonadenomas: assessment of washout at delayed contrast-enhanced CT. Radiology 1998;207: 369–75.
20. Peña CS, Boland GW, Hahn PF, et al. Characterization of indeterminate (lipid-poor) adrenal masses: use of washout characteristics at contrast-enhanced CT. Radiology 2000;217:798–802.
21. Caoili EM, Korobkin M, Francis IR, et al. Adrenal masses: characterization with combined unenhanced and delayed enhanced CT. Radiology 2002;222:629–33.
22. Blake MA, Kalra MK, Sweeney AT, et al. Distinguishing benign from malignant adrenal masses: multi-detector row CT protocol with 10-minute delay. Radiology 2006;238:578–85.
23. Caoili EM, Korobkin M, Francis IR, et al. Delayed enhanced CT of lipid-poor adrenal adenomas. AJR Am J Roentgenol 2000;175:1411–5.
24. Mitchell DG, Crovello M, Matteucci T, et al. Benign adrenocortical masses: diagnosis with chemical shift MR imaging. Radiology 1992;185:345–51.
25. Outwater EK, Siegelman ES, Radecki PD, et al. Distinction between benign and malignant adrenal masses: value of T1-weighted chemical-shift MR imaging. AJR Am J Roentgenol 1995;165:579–83.
26. Mayo-smith WW, Boland GW, Noto RB, et al. State-of-the-art adrenal imaging. Radiographics 2001;21: 995–1012.
27. Fujiyoshi F, Nakajo M, Fukukura Y, et al. Characterization of adrenal tumors by chemical shift fast low-angle shot MR imaging: comparison of four

methods of quantitative evaluation. AJR Am J Roentgenol 2003;180:1649–57.

28. Outwater EK, Siegelman ES, Huang AB, et al. Adrenal masses: correlation between CT attenuation value and chemical shift ratio at MR imaging with in-phase and opposed-phase sequences. Radiology 1996;200:749–52.

29. Mayo-Smith WW, Lee MJ, McNicholas MM, et al. Characterization of adrenal masses (<5cm) by use of chemical shift MR imaging: observer performance versus quantitative measures. AJR Am J Roentgenol 1995;165:91–5.

30. Gabriel H, Pizzitola V, McComb EN, et al. Adrenal lesions with heterogenous suppression on chemical shift imaging: clinical implications. J Magn Reson Imaging 2004;19:308–16.

31. Israel GM, Korobkin M, Wang C, et al. Comparison of unenhanced CT and chemical shift MRI in evaluating lipid-rich adrenal adenomas. AJR Am J Roentgenol 2004;183:215–9.

32. Haider MA, Ghai S, Jhaveri K, et al. Chemical shift MR imaging of hyperattenuating (>10 HU) adrenal masses: does it still have a role? Radiology 2004;231:711–6.

33. Park BK, Kim CK, Kim B, et al. Comparison of delayed enhanced CT and chemical shift MR for evaluating hyperattenuating incidental adrenal masses. Radiology 2007;243:760–5.

34. Krestin GP, Steinbrich W, Friedmann G. Adrenal masses: evaluation with fast gradient-echo MR imaging and Gd-DTPA-enhanced dynamic studies. Radiology 1989;171:675–80.

35. Dunnick NR, Korobkin M. Imaging of adrenal incidentalomas: current status. AJR Am J Roentgenol 2002;179:559–68.

36. Metser U, Miller E, Lerman H, et al. 18F-FDG PET/CT in the evaluation of adrenal masses. J Nucl Med 2006;47:32–7.

37. Kumar R, Xiu Y, Yu JQ, et al. 18F-FDG PET in evaluation of adrenal lesions in patients with lung cancer. J Nucl Med 2004;45:2058–62.

38. Chong S, Lee KS, Kim HY, et al. Integrated PET-CT for the characterization of adrenal gland lesions in cancer patients: diagnostic efficacy and interpretation pitfalls. Radiographics 2006;26:1811–26.

39. Boland GW, Blake MA, Holakere NS, et al. PET/CT for the characterization of adrenal masses in patients with cancer: qualitative vs quantitative accuracy in 150 consecutive patients. AJR Am J Roentgenol 2009;192:956–62.

40. Paulsen SD, Nghiem HV, Korobkin M, et al. Changing role of imaging-guided percutaneous biopsy of adrenal masses: evaluation of 50 adrenal biopsies. AJR Am J Roentgenol 2004;182:1033–7.

41. Silverman SG, Mueller PR, Pinkney LP, et al. Predictive value of image-guided adrenal biopsy: analysis of results of 101 biopsies. Radiology 1993;187:715–8.

42. Welch TJ, Sheedy PF II, Stephens DH, et al. Percutaneous adrenal biopsy: review of a 10-year experience. Radiology 1994;193:341–4.

The Incidental Renal Mass

Gary M. Israel, MD[a],*, Stuart G. Silverman, MD[b]

KEYWORDS
- Renal mass • Renal cell carcinoma • Renal cyst
- Incidental • Angiomyolipoma

Incidental renal masses are extremely common.[1,2] Although most represent benign renal cysts, not all incidental renal masses are benign.[2] Most renal cell carcinomas are discovered incidentally when an imaging examination is performed to evaluate a nonrenal complaint.[3–6] Therefore, differentiating incidental benign renal masses from those that are potentially malignant is important. There are well-established, time-tested, image-based criteria that can be used to diagnose most renal masses definitively.[7–33] However, some renal masses remain indeterminate even after a thorough evaluation with imaging. This article discusses the evaluation, diagnosis, and treatment options of the incidental renal mass.

RENAL PSEUDOTUMORS: CONFIRMATION OF AN ABNORMAL FINDING

When encountering any renal mass, it is necessary to first determine whether the detected abnormality represents a pseudotumor, a masslike finding that mimics a neoplasm. Renal pseudotumors are caused by a variety of conditions including congenital anomalies (prominent renal columns of Bertin, dromedary humps), inflammatory masses (focal pyelonephritis, chronic renal abscess, autoimmune disease), vascular structures (renal artery aneurysm or arteriovenous fistula), or abnormalities relating to trauma or hemorrhage. Although some renal pseudotumors require treatment, they are treated differently from neoplasms and therefore their recognition is important to ensure proper management. If they

are not first excluded when evaluating a renal masslike finding, the application of image-based criteria used to evaluate renal masses could lead to an incorrect diagnosis. For example, enhancement is often used to support the diagnosis of a neoplasm, but enhancement can be found in infectious and other inflammatory conditions, aneurysms, and vascular malformations. Key radiologic features to support an inflammatory cause include ill-defined margins and perinephric stranding (Fig. 1). Aneurysms and vascular malformations enhance similarly to nearby vasculature; in the case of a vascular malformation, hypertrophy of the ipsilateral renal artery and arteriovenous shunting may be present. In most cases, careful evaluation of computed tomography (CT) or magnetic resonance (MR) imaging, combined with the clinical presentation and a familiarity with this group of masses, should reveal the correct diagnosis.

CLINICAL HISTORY AND DEMOGRAPHIC INFORMATION

Clinical history and demographic patient information are noncontributory in diagnosing an incidental renal mass in most cases. Most patients with renal cell carcinoma are asymptomatic and the tumor is serendipitously found on an imaging study performed for a nonrenal complaint.[3–6] History can be helpful in differentiating a masslike inflammatory process of the kidney (pseudotumor) from a renal neoplasm. A history of flank pain, fever, and pyuria are supportive of pyelonephritis, and not a neoplasm

[a] Department of Radiology, Smilow Cancer Hospital, Yale University School of Medicine, 2nd Floor North Pavillion, Room 2–245, New Haven, CT 06520, USA
[b] Department of Radiology, Brigham and Women's Hospital, Harvard Medical School, 75 Francis Street, Boston, MA 02115, USA
* Corresponding author.
E-mail address: gary.israel@yale.edu

Radiol Clin N Am 49 (2011) 369–383
doi:10.1016/j.rcl.2010.10.007

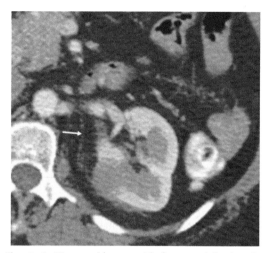

Fig. 1. A 48-year-old man with fever and flank pain. Axial contrast-enhanced CT image shows a 2.3-cm mass in the left kidney. The mass has ill-defined margins with the kidney and there is mild perinephric stranding (*arrow*). Combined with the clinical history of fever and flank pain, the findings are consistent with focal pyelonephritis. The patient was successfully treated with antibiotics. Follow-up CT scan (not shown) showed complete resolution.

(see **Fig. 1**). However, these signs and symptoms do not exclude the diagnosis of a neoplasm. Patient demographics and a specific imaging appearance may be helpful in interpreting some renal masses and suggesting appropriate management. For instance, angiomyolipoma with minimal fat and multilocular cystic nephroma, both discussed in detail later, are more common in women and have typical imaging characteristics, but cannot be diagnosed with certainty using imaging alone.

ENHANCEMENT OF RENAL MASSES

Once pseudotumors are excluded, mass enhancement indicates a neoplasm. Renal mass enhancement is affected by multiple factors: the amount and rate of the contrast material injected, scan delay, and the vascularity of the mass. Highly vascular tumors show marked enhancement, whereas hypovascular tumors show minimal enhancement. Enhancement is assessed on CT imaging by comparing the attenuation of the mass, measured in Hounsfield units (HU), before and after intravenous (IV) contrast material administration. There is no universally agreed specific value that can be used as a cutoff for differentiating nonenhancing fluid from enhancing soft tissue. We use a threshold of 20 HU to indicate definitive enhancement within a renal mass, values of 10 to 19 HU as equivocal for enhancement, and values of less than 10 HU as indicating no enhancement.[7]

The accuracy of attenuation values are dependent on multiple factors, including patient size, renal mass size, size and placement of the region of interest, CT technique, partial volume averaging, and CT scanner type and manufacturer.[8–11] In our opinion, these are time-tested values and ranges and represent a practical approach to determining enhancement.

There is no unanimously accepted way of determining renal mass enhancement with MR imaging. Methods currently used include image subtraction,[12] calculating percent enhancement using arbitrary signal intensity units,[12,13] and subjective comparison of unenhanced and contrast-enhanced images. Although a subjective comparison of unenhanced and contrast-enhanced images may be useful in cases of obvious enhancement in hypervascular tumors, enhancement may be difficult (or impossible) to detect in hypovascular tumors and in masses that are hyperintense on unenhanced T1-weighted images.

CYSTIC RENAL MASSES

Cystic renal masses are the most common masses in the kidney, with most being benign simple cysts.[2] Simple cysts are defined as having a hairline-thin wall, no septa or calcification, and being filled with simple fluid that measures 0 to 20 HU. There are no soft tissue components within simple cysts, they do not enhance after the administration of IV contrast, and they are considered benign.[14] When a cystic renal mass contains material that is higher in attenuation than simple fluid (>20 HU), 1 or more septa, calcifications, thickened walls or septa, or enhancing soft tissue components, it cannot be considered a simple cyst. The Bosniak renal cyst classification system has been used worldwide in evaluating cystic renal masses for the past 25 years.[14–18] Cystic renal masses are classified into 5 groups based on CT findings: categories I, II, IIF, III, and IV.[19–22]

Category I masses are simple cysts using the criteria listed earlier and are always benign. Category II masses are minimally complicated cysts that can be reliably considered as benign. They may contain a few (generally 1 or 2) hairline-thin septa in which perceived (not measurable) enhancement may be appreciated. The wall or septa may contain fine calcifications or a short segment of slightly thickened smooth calcification (**Fig. 2**).

Hyperdense or hyperattenuating cysts are also included in category II. These masses were initially described as containing attenuations greater than renal parenchyma (typically 40–90 HU), but the attenuation criterion has been expanded to

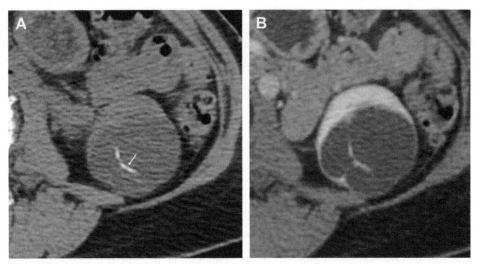

Fig. 2. A 63-year-old woman with a Bosniak category II renal cyst. Unenhanced (*A*) and contrast-enhanced (*B*) axial CT images show a cystic left renal mass that contains a few hairline-thin septa in which thin curvilinear calcification is present (*arrow*). There is no measurable enhancement within the mass and its wall is hairline thin. The mass is consistent with a category II mass (benign). Note the slight puckering in of the wall of the mass at the point where septa insert on the wall. This puckering should not be mistaken for enhancing soft tissue components within the mass.

include masses with attenuations greater than 20 HU.[7] To diagnose a hyperattenuating cyst with confidence, the mass must be small (≤3 cm), well circumscribed, homogeneously hyperattenuating (even on a narrow window setting), and must not enhance (Fig. 3). Homogeneity is an important feature; high-attenuation fluid within a renal mass can mask small regions of enhancement. Therefore, it is important to obtain multiple attenuation measurements of varying sizes throughout the lesion to ensure that the mass is homogeneous, and that no portion of the mass enhances. To our knowledge, there is only a single case report in the literature that fulfils the criteria for a hyperattenuating cyst and was subsequently proved to represent a renal cell carcinoma.[23] At pathology, the mass was cystic and contained only a single layer of neoplastic cells in its wall. Nonetheless, it is our opinion that small (≤3 cm) homogeneously high-attenuation nonenhancing cystic renal masses, are reliably considered benign and do not need further evaluation. Hyperattenuating cysts may be diagnosed by unenhanced CT alone; a recent study showed

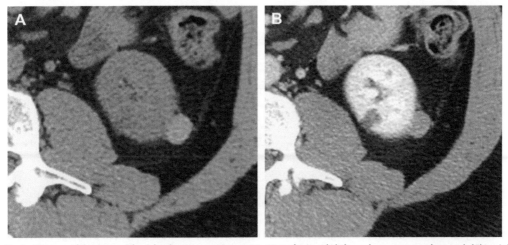

Fig. 3. A 45-year-old man with a high-attenuation cyst. Unenhanced (*A*) and contrast-enhanced (*B*) axial CT images show a 1.3-cm nonenhancing hyperattenuating homogeneous mass in the left kidney that measures 74 HU on the unenhanced examination. This mass is consistent with a hyperattenuating cyst (Bosniak category II). Note the other small low-attenuation lesions in the kidney that are likely a cluster of benign cysts.

that a renal mass with homogeneous attenuation greater than 70 HU on an unenhanced CT had a greater than 99% probability of being benign (Fig. 3).[24] Although additional studies are necessary, it seems that some high-attenuation cysts can be diagnosed as benign without additional imaging or contrast material administration.

Overall, Bosniak category II renal masses are reliably considered benign. The clinical significance of case reports of category II masses that were found to be malignant,[16,23,25,34] some with only a single microscopic foci of malignant cells in the wall,[23] is unclear. Some of the reports did not describe fully the imaging findings, and it is possible that the lesions were incorrectly categorized. Even if they were appropriately categorized, the number of malignant category II renal masses is extremely small compared with the number of benign category II masses. It is likely that those masses described in the cases reports were low-grade (Fuhrman grade I) renal cell carcinomas. Therefore, a medically appropriate and practical approach is to consider all category II masses benign.

Category IIF masses (F for follow-up)[20,21,26,27] have more features than those defined for a category II mass. Category IIF lesions are likely benign but require follow-up imaging to show stability. These masses may contain multiple hairline-thin septa and a slightly thickened smooth wall or septum in which perceived enhancement (not measurable enhancement) is present (see Fig. 4). Category IIF renal masses may contain thick or nodular calcification, but there should not be any enhancing soft tissue elements.[21] Category IIF includes nonenhancing hyperattenuating renal masses that measure greater than 3 cm or are completely intrarenal. Category IIF masses should be followed for morphologic changes, such as development of septa or wall thickening. Growth is not a useful determinant of malignancy because simple benign cysts may grow and renal cell carcinomas may not.[20,35–39] Therefore, growth is not a feature of the Bosniak renal cyst classification. Morphologic changes, such as septa or wall thickening or new areas of enhancement, suggest malignancy. Because lack of morphologic change with time suggests a benign diagnosis, following category IIF masses is appropriate. In a study of 42 patients with category IIF masses, only 2 patients' masses showed progressive septa thickening on follow-up examinations and were diagnosed as renal cell carcinoma 1.5 and 3 years after the initial CT scan.[20] The recommended interval for follow-up examinations is to obtain a CT scan or MR imaging examination at 6 and 12 months, followed by yearly examinations for a minimum of 5 years.[20] However, there is no known time interval of stability that can be used to diagnose a renal mass as benign with complete certainty. However, if a Bosniak category IIF lesion

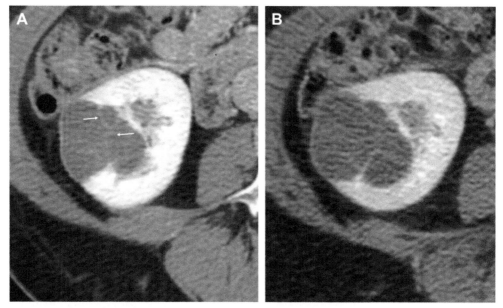

Fig. 4. A 54-year-old woman with a benign complicated renal cyst. (A) Contrast-enhanced CT image shows a 2.5-cm cystic right renal mass that contains multiple thin septa (arrows), consistent with a Bosniak category IIF cyst. There are no solid enhancing components. (B) Contrast-enhanced CT image obtained 3 years after the examination in (A) shows that the mass may be slightly larger but that there no other morphologic changes in the appearance of the mass, suggesting a benign cause. Further follow-up examinations will be performed to ensure benignity.

has not significantly changed morphologically in a period of 5 years, it is likely benign.[20]

Category III cysts are truly indeterminate masses because they have a reasonable probability of being benign or malignant. Imaging features include a thickened wall or septa that show measurable enhancement (**Figs. 5** and **6**).[19,28] Benign masses in this category include acute and chronically infected cysts, hemorrhagic cysts (often secondary to trauma), benign multilocular cysts, benign multiseptated cysts, and cystic neoplasms such as multilocular cystic nephroma. Malignant masses in this category include cystic renal cell carcinoma. Initially, it was estimated that approximately half of category III masses were benign and the other half were malignant. Recent studies have shown a wide range (31%–100%) of these masses to be malignant.[15,40] This wide variation may be attributed to radiologists' experience in interpreting renal mass imaging and the philosophy and practice of referring urologists caring for the patient. Since category IIF was introduced, we believe that most category III renal masses have been malignant; benign category III masses that previously were operated on are now being followed (category IIF) with a subsequent greater percentage of malignant category III masses remaining.

Most category III masses are treated by surgical resection to ensure that a malignancy is not missed. This approach leads to some benign lesions unnecessarily being removed. The number of benign category III masses that are removed can be reduced by always considering benign diagnoses that can be treated nonsurgically, such as renal abscesses and some hemorrhagic cysts. Percutaneous biopsy is of limited value, but may be helpful in patients who have comorbidities that place them at risk for surgery.[40,41] If a malignant result is achieved; this allows the surgery to proceed with confidence. If a definitive diagnosis of a benign entity is obtained, surgery can be avoided. However, unless a specific benign result is obtained, other negative results (eg, nonspecific biopsy specimens containing inflammatory cells) should be viewed with skepticism.[29] Biopsy can be difficult because Bosniak category III masses typically contain no soft tissue nodules; there is less tumor to sample, and hence the possibility of sampling error. Therefore, it should be emphasized to the patient and referring physician that a negative biopsy result may not be definitive.[29]

Category IV cysts are malignant masses until proved otherwise and therefore require surgical removal. Imaging features include those described in category III with the presence of nodular enhancement within the mass or adjacent to its wall (**Fig. 7**). The probability of such a mass being malignant is close to 100%.

CYSTIC RENAL MASS SIZE AS A FACTOR

Size is not a good predictor of malignancy in cystic renal masses because small cystic masses may be malignant and large ones can be benign. In our experience, the smaller the cystic lesion, the more likely it is benign, and very small (<1 cm) cystic renal mass are almost always benign. This finding is important because subcentimeter cystic masses

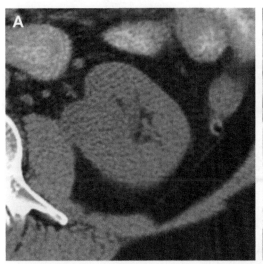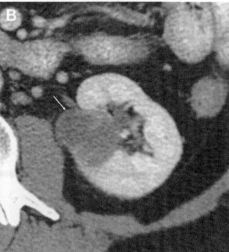

Fig. 5. A 47-year-old man with a Bosniak category III renal mass. Axial contrast-enhanced CT image shows a 3.3-cm mass in the left kidney that contains a thickened wall in which measurable enhancement could be measured (*arrow*). The mass is consistent with a Bosniak category III mass. The patient underwent partial nephrectomy and a renal cell carcinoma was diagnosed at pathology.

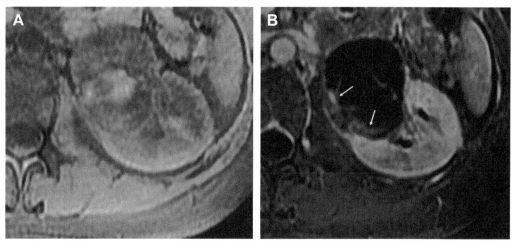

Fig. 6. A 33-year-old woman with a category III cystic renal mass. Unenhanced fat-suppressed T1-weighted image (A) and postcontrast fat-suppressed T1-weighted image (subtraction image obtained by subtracting the unenhanced image in (A) from a contrast-enhanced image [not shown]) (B) shows a 4.5-cm cystic mass with irregular and thickened enhancing septa (arrows), consistent with a Bosniak category III mass. Renal cell carcinoma was diagnosed at pathology.

are more difficult to characterize compared with larger cystic masses, because their morphologic features are not as evident. With the technological advances in CT during the past 20 years, more cystic-appearing masses measuring less than 1 cm are being detected in the kidneys. Many of these masses cannot be characterized accurately because of their small size. However, the probability of a small cystic lesion being benign is extremely high. Therefore, as Bosniak recommended in the

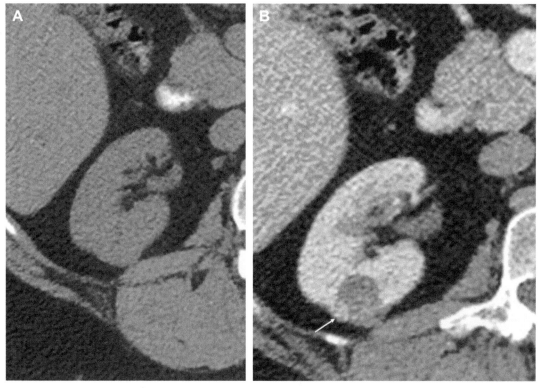

Fig. 7. A 74-year-old man with a complex cystic renal mass. Unenhanced (A) and contrast-enhanced (B) axial CT images show a 1.7-cm cystic mass in the right kidney that contains a solid enhancing nodule along its wall (arrow). This is consistent with a Bosniak category IV mass, a renal cell carcinoma was diagnosed at pathology.

past, we believe that a small (<1 cm) cystic-appearing mass that is homogeneously low in attenuation and without septa, nodularity, or calcification can be diagnosed as a benign cyst.[30,42]

SOLID RENAL MASSES

A solid renal mass is best defined as a mass with little or no fluid components, and usually consists predominantly of enhancing soft tissue. As detailed earlier, after excluding pseudotumors, such as inflammatory causes, and vascular anomalies and aneurysms, a solid renal mass should be considered a renal neoplasm. Most solid renal neoplasms in adults are renal cell carcinoma and surgery is recommended. However, many small (≤3 cm) solid renal masses are benign.[43] Benign diagnoses typically encountered at surgery for what was believed to be renal carcinoma include oncocytomas and angiomyolipomas. Oncocytomas are benign tumors that historically have been resected because they could not be distinguished from renal cell carcinoma with confidence. As a result, most are still resected; however, percutaneous biopsy can be used to render a confident diagnosis in some cases, and this is discussed later.[29] Most angiomyolipomas can be diagnosed by showing with CT or MR imaging the presence of fat in a noncalcified renal mass. As a result, angiomyolipomas that are resected today are typically those that contain little or no fat.

It is also necessary to diagnose those malignant renal neoplasms that do not require surgery (eg, lymphoma and metastatic disease). A combination of clinical history and the imaging findings may allow these masses to be diagnosed. However, in some cases percutaneous biopsy may be required. In the setting of an extrarenal malignancy that is known to metastasize to the kidney, the mass may represent a primary renal malignancy or metastatic disease. In patients with a history of extrarenal malignancy, 50% to 85% of solitary solid renal masses are metastatic.[44,45] Therefore, a metastasis cannot be diagnosed presumptively, and other benign and malignant primary renal neoplasms need to be considered.[31] In patients with widespread metastatic disease, this differentiation may not be necessary clinically but, in patients with an extrarenal neoplasm without metastatic disease, percutaneous biopsy may help diagnose the mass.[29,31]

When multiple non–fat-containing solid renal masses are identified in a patient without a history of extrarenal malignancy, the most likely diagnoses are multifocal renal cell carcinoma or multiple oncocytomas (which may or may not be part of a hereditary syndrome).[46–48] In these cases, renal mass biopsy is usually performed for diagnosis before making management decisions because patients with multifocal renal cell carcinoma are typically treated more aggressively than those with multiple oncocytomas.[32,33,42] In patients with a history of an extrarenal malignancy (especially lung cancer and lymphoma) who are found to have multiple solid renal masses, metastatic disease (in addition to multifocal renal cell carcinoma and multiple oncocytomas) needs to be considered and renal mass biopsy is suggested for differentiation.

As mentioned earlier, although solitary solid renal masses are frequently renal cell carcinoma, many also represent benign masses (angiomyolipoma and oncocytoma), particularly when they are small. Most angiomyolipomas can be diagnosed with CT or MR imaging by showing regions of fat within a mass.[49] Some angiomyolipomas contain very small quantities of fat that can be overlooked if the mass is not carefully evaluated (Fig. 8).[50,51] Meticulous evaluation of all solid renal masses for the presence of fat is imperative to avoid recommending surgical excision of an angiomyolipoma. When a small amount of fat is suspected in a renal mass, an unenhanced CT scan with thin sections combined with a pixel analysis is the most sensitive test to confirm this.[50–52] MR imaging using T1-weighted sequences with and without frequency-selective fat suppression or chemical shift imaging can also be used.[53] Approximately 5% of angiomyolipomas do not contain fat that can be seen at imaging, and the differentiation from other renal neoplasms is not possible with CT or MR imaging. These masses, referred to as angiomyolipoma with minimal fat,[51] are often small, hyperattenuating on an unenhanced CT examination (attenuation > unenhanced renal tissue) and homogeneously enhance with contrast material (Fig. 9).[51,54] However, these findings are not specific enough to make a confident diagnosis of an angiomyolipoma, and other tumors, such as papillary renal cell carcinoma, metanephric adenoma, oncocytoma and leiomyoma, may have a similar appearance.[33,55,56]

MR imaging may be useful when an angiomyolipoma with minimal fat is suspected on CT. Angiomyolipomas with minimal fat contain a lot of smooth muscle and are therefore typically hypointense on T2-weighted images[51,57] compared with clear cell renal cell carcinoma (the most common subtype of renal cell carcinoma), which is typically hyperintense on T2-weighted images.[58–61] Therefore, if a solid renal mass shows high attenuation on an unenhanced CT scan, homogeneously enhances, and is hypointense on T2-weighted images, an angiomyolipoma with minimal fat is a possible diagnosis, especially if the patient is

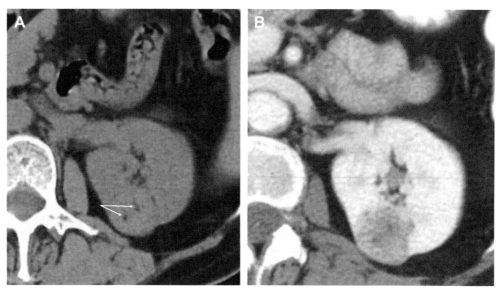

Fig. 8. A 65-year-old woman with an angiomyolipoma (AML) that contains a small amount of fat. Unenhanced (A) and contrast-enhanced (B) CT images show a 2-cm solid enhancing mass in the left kidney. A small amount of fat can be identified on the unenhanced image (arrows), which is diagnostic of AML. However, it is possible that small amounts of fat can be overlooked if the examination is not carefully evaluated, and a renal cell carcinoma may be incorrectly diagnosed.

a woman. However, this is not diagnostic because other renal masses may have similar appearances. Specifically, papillary renal cell carcinoma may also enhance homogeneously and is typically hypointense on T2-weighted sequences.[59,62] Therefore, when imaging suggests the diagnosis of angiomyolipoma with minimal fat but cannot exclude

papillary renal cell carcinoma, renal mass biopsy is suggested to differentiate between these 2 entities.[29]

Oncocytoma is a benign solid renal mass that cannot be differentiated from renal cell carcinoma by imaging. Although a central scar and homogeneous enhancement at CT or MR imaging are

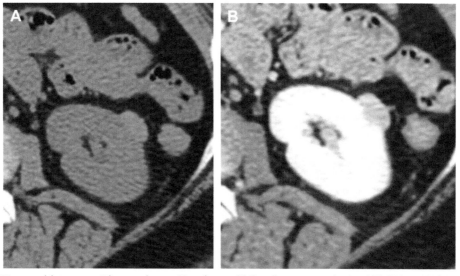

Fig. 9. A 42-year-old woman with a renal mass. Unenhanced (A) and contrast-enhanced (B) CT images show a 1.2-cm solid homogeneously enhancing exophytic left renal mass that is high in attenuation on the unenhanced image. Although the imaging findings are not specific, the findings are suggestive of an AML with minimal fat. A percutaneous biopsy was taken from the mass and an AML was diagnosed.

suggestive of oncocytoma, these findings are not specific and a tissue diagnosis is necessary to differentiate oncocytoma from renal cell carcinomas that have also been reported to display these findings. Percutaneous biopsy has recently been used to diagnose small oncocytomas; the appearance of an oncocytoma on biopsy specimens can be characteristic and the diagnosis further corroborated using special immunocytochemical stains. However, biopsy is not definitive in all cases, because some renal cell carcinomas have oncocytic features, and surgical resection may be needed to make a definitive diagnosis.[29,63]

SOLID RENAL MASS SIZE AS A FACTOR

A study of 2770 surgically removed solid renal masses showed that 12.8% of the masses were benign, of which almost all were oncocytomas and angiomyolipomas.[43] When all renal masses were stratified according to size, 46% of masses less than 1 cm were benign, as were 22% of those that were between 1 and 2.9 cm, and 20% of those that were between 3 and 3.9 cm. Smaller solid renal masses are therefore more likely to be benign than larger masses. Although there are limited data regarding the natural history of small (≤3 cm) solid renal masses, they are usually low grade with a slow growth rate. Similar growth rates have been shown for both benign and malignant small solid renal masses.[5,64–68] Some small solid renal masses may not grow at all. In one meta-analysis, 30% of small (≤3 cm) solid renal masses did not grow during a 23- to 39-month observation interval.[66] Another study showed that the chance of malignancy in a renal mass that is stable in size was approximately the same as an enlarging mass, 83% versus 89%, respectively.[38] However, some small renal cell carcinomas can be histologically aggressive,[69] grow quickly,[66] and metastasize early. Therefore, it is difficult to predict the clinical behavior of a renal mass based on size or histology alone.

IMAGING MODALITIES AND TECHNIQUES

It is common to find incidental renal masses when imaging the abdomen, and most are simple cysts. If the mass does not seem to represent a simple cyst, a CT or MR imaging examination designed to evaluate renal masses is usually necessary. Exceptions include masses that can be characterized on the initial study, such as obvious renal cell carcinoma, angiomyolipomas that show fat, and some benign complicated renal cysts (Bosniak category II). The imaging modality used to characterize a renal mass is dependent on the preference and experience of the radiologist and urologist. In some cases, ultrasound can be used to characterize a renal mass. Ultrasound is best used to characterize simple cysts; benign, minimally complicated cysts that are well imaged with ultrasound may not need additional imaging. CT and MR imaging are the most frequently used modalities to characterize a known renal mass. Although it this article does not review the CT and MR imaging techniques used to characterize renal masses in detail, it is necessary to perform both examinations with 3- to 5-mm sections before and after the administration of IV contrast material.

Follow-up imaging can be used as part of an observational strategy of renal masses, most recently referred to as active surveillance. It is frequently used in patients with renal masses that would have been surgical removed, but who are not surgical candidates because of surgical comorbidities or limited life expectancy. Follow-up imaging is used to determine interval growth of the mass. Any imaging modality that can be used to show the mass clearly enough to obtain accurate measurements is suitable. Unenhanced imaging may be adequate in follow-up imaging. In cases of Bosniak category IIF cysts, follow-up imaging with and without contrast is necessary because morphologic characteristics and enhancement of the mass is needed in addition to lesion size. Therefore, protocols used to characterize a renal mass (CT or MR imaging with and without IV contrast material) should be used when following Bosniak category IIF masses.

MANAGEMENT RECOMMENDATIONS

Management decisions are dependent on many factors, including imaging findings, patient age, life expectancy, comorbidities, available treatment options, and patient preference. A 3-cm non–fat-containing solid mass that would typically be surgically removed in the general population would require an alternate management strategy, such as follow-up imaging or ablation, in a patient at high surgical risk. Because each patient is unique, it is impossible to develop management schemes that would be appropriate for all patients. The management of each patient needs to be individualized, and appropriate management should consider imaging findings in addition to clinical factors.

RECOMMENDATIONS IN PATIENTS WITH CYSTIC RENAL MASSES
General Population

The Bosniak renal cyst classification is recommended as the guideline for management in the general population (Table 1). Although renal

Table 1
Management recommendations for patients with an incidental cystic renal mass

Bosniak Category	Appearance — Imaging Features	Recommendation — General Population	Recommendation — Comorbidities or Limited Life Expectancy
I[a]	Hairline-thin wall; no septa, calcifications, or solid components; water attenuation; no enhancement	Ignore	Ignore
II	Few hairline-thin septa with or without perceived (not measurable) enhancement; fine calcification or short segment of slightly thickened calcification in the wall or septa; homogeneously high-attenuating masses(≤3 cm) that are sharply marginated and do not enhance	Ignore	Ignore
IIF	Multiple hairline-thin septa with or without perceived (not measurable) enhancement, minimal smooth thickening of wall or septa that may show perceived (not measurable) enhancement, calcification may be thick and nodular but no measurable enhancement present; no enhancing soft tissue components; intrarenal nonenhancing high-attenuation renal masses (>3 cm)	Observe[b,c]	Observe[b] or ignore[d]
III	Thickened irregular or smooth walls or septa, with measurable enhancement	Surgery[e]	Surgery[e] or observe[b]
IV	Criteria of category III but also containing enhancing soft tissue components adjacent to or separate from the wall or septa	Surgery[e]	Surgery[e] or observe[b]

Note: These recommendations are to be followed only if nonneoplastic causes of a renal mass (eg, infections) have been excluded; see text for details. The recommendations are offered as general guidelines and do not necessarily apply to all patients.

[a] When a mass smaller than 1 cm has the appearance of a simple cyst, further work-up is not likely to yield useful information.

[b] CT or MR imaging at 6 and 12 months, then yearly for 5 years; interval and duration of observation may be varied (eg, longer intervals may be chosen if the mass is unchanged; longer duration may be chosen for greater assurance).

[c] In selected patients, (eg, young) early surgical intervention may be considered, particularly if a minimally invasive approach (eg, laparoscopic partial nephrectomy) can be used.

[d] Cystic masses 1.5 cm or smaller that are not clearly simple cysts, or that cannot be characterized completely, may not require further evaluation in patients with comorbidities and in patients with limited life expectancy.

[e] Surgical options include open or laparoscopic nephrectomy and partial nephrectomy; each provides a tissue diagnosis. Open, laparoscopic, and percutaneous ablation may be considered where available, but biopsy would be needed to achieve a tissue diagnosis. Long-term (5- or 10-year) results of ablation are not yet known.

mass size is generally not a part of the Bosniak classification, renal masses that measure less than 1 cm and seem to represent simple cysts (low attenuating without septa, nodularity, calcification, or enhancement), can be presumed to be benign and do not need to be further evaluated.[30] Although the true nature of these masses is unclear, it is reasonable to report that they are too small to diagnose definitively, but are statistically likely to represent benign renal cysts.

Patients with Limited Life Expectancy or Significant Comorbidity

Similarly to cystic masses in the general population, the Bosniak classification can be used, but with a less aggressive approach (see Table 1). In addition, incidental indeterminate renal masses measuring up to 1.5 cm when they are first discovered need not be further evaluated in patients with comorbidities that limit life expectancy.[30] This is based on the idea that most of these masses will be benign cysts or slow-growing neoplasms.[36,70,71]

RECOMMENDATIONS IN PATIENTS WITH SOLID RENAL MASSES
General Population

Solid renal masses are more likely to be malignant than cystic masses and a more aggressive approach is recommended (Table 2). With the exception of angiomyolipoma, benign and malignant solid renal masses cannot be differentiated with imaging, and histologic diagnosis is suggested. Similarly to cystic masses, masses smaller than 1 cm that seem solid are challenging from a management perspective. Despite state-of-the art CT and MR imaging techniques, correctly diagnosing the mass as solid is difficult, given their small size. Even if the mass can be correctly characterized as solid, there is as much as a 46 % chance that the mass would be benign.[43] Therefore, when a mass in the kidney measures less than 1 cm and has features that suggest it is solid, it is reasonable to follow the mass with serial imaging (initially 3–6 months and then yearly), until the mass reaches 1 cm in size. At this time, the mass should be of sufficient size to be able to be further characterized.

Patients with Limited Life Expectancy or Comorbidities

In patients with limited life expectancy or comorbidities, a less aggressive approach may be used from that of the general population (Table 3), especially for small (≤3 cm) renal masses because they are more likely to be benign and are less aggressive than larger masses. These masses can be observed with serial imaging in lieu of surgery. In the past, Bosniak has suggested observation in patients with solid masses smaller than 1.5 cm because most small renal cell carcinomas grow

Table 2
Management recommendations for an incidental solid renal mass in patients in the general population

Mass Size (cm)	Probable Diagnosis	Recommendation	Comment
Large (>3)	Renal cell carcinoma[a]	Surgery[b]	Angiomyolipoma with minimal fat, oncocytoma, other benign neoplasms may be found at surgery
Small (1–3)	Renal cell carcinoma[a]	Surgery[b]	If hyperattenuating, and homogeneously enhancing, consider MR imaging and percutaneous biopsy to diagnose angiomyolipoma with minimal fat
Very small (<1)	Renal cell carcinoma, oncocytoma, angiomyolipoma[c]	Observe until 1 cm[d]	Thin (≤3 mm) sections help confirm enhancement

Note: These recommendations are best followed after nonneoplastic causes of a renal mass (eg, infections) have been excluded; see text for details. The recommendations are offered as general guidelines and do not necessarily apply to all patients.

[a] Provided there is no detectable fat by CT or MR imaging using protocols designed to evaluate renal masses.

[b] Surgical options include open or laparoscopic nephrectomy and partial nephrectomy; both provide a tissue diagnosis. Open, laparoscopic, and percutaneous ablation may be considered where available, but biopsy would be needed to achieve a tissue diagnosis. Long-term (5- or 10-year) results of ablation are not yet known.

[c] Benign entities are more likely in small renal masses than large ones.

[d] CT or MR imaging at 3 to 6 months, and 12 months, then yearly; interval and duration of observation may be varied (eg, shorter intervals if the mass is enlarging).

Table 3
Management recommendations for an incidental solid renal mass in patients with limited life expectancy or comorbidities that increase the risk of treatment

Mass Size (cm)	Probable Diagnosis	Recommendation	Comment
Large (>3)	Renal cell carcinoma[a]	Surgery[b] or observe	Angiomyolipoma with minimal fat, oncocytoma, other benign neoplasms may be found at surgery; Biopsy can be used preoperatively to confirm renal cell carcinoma
Small (1–3)	Renal cell carcinoma[a]	Surgery[b] or observe	If hyperattenuating, and homogeneously enhancing, consider MR imaging and percutaneous biopsy to diagnose angiomyolipoma with minimal fat
Very small (<1)	Renal cell carcinoma, oncocytoma, angiomyolipoma[c]	Observe until 1.5 cm[d]	Thin (≤3 mm) sections help confirm enhancement

Note: These recommendations are best followed after nonneoplastic causes of a renal mass (eg, infections) have been excluded; see text for details. The recommendations are offered as general guidelines and do not necessarily apply to all patients.

[a] Provided there is no detectable fat by CT or MR imaging using protocols designed to evaluate renal masses.

[b] Surgical options include open or laparoscopic nephrectomy and partial nephrectomy; both provide a tissue diagnosis. Open, laparoscopic, and percutaneous ablation may be considered where available, but biopsy would be needed to achieve a tissue diagnosis. Long-term (5- or 10-year) results of ablation are not yet known.

[c] Benign entities are more likely in small renal masses than large ones.

[d] CT or MR imaging at 3 to 6 months, and 12 months, then yearly; interval of observation may be varied (eg, shorter intervals if the mass is enlarging); duration of observation may be individualized. Observation may be considered for a solid renal mass of any size in a patient with limited life expectancy, or comorbidities that increase the risk of treatment, particularly when the mass is small. It may be safe to observe a solid renal mass beyond 1.5 cm; however, there are insufficient data to provide definitive recommendations on the risks and benefits of observation.

slowly.[35–37] An expert panel commission of the American College of Radiology also supports a wait-and-see approach for renal masses of 1.5 cm or less in the elderly.[72] Because solid renal masses represent renal cell carcinoma in most cases, and are only curable when they are confined to the kidney, a decision to observe should be made carefully.

Options for the treatment of renal masses are increasing. Historically, radical nephrectomy was the standard of care for patients with renal cell carcinoma, both solid and cystic types. Partial nephrectomy is now recommended for T1a masses (organ-confined masses ≤4 cm).[73] Minimally invasive techniques, including laparoscopic partial nephrectomy and laparoscopic and percutaneous ablation, may be considered, particularly for patients with comorbidities.

SUMMARY

Incidental renal masses are extremely common. Although most have benign causes, some are renal cell carcinoma. The guidelines we recommend are an attempt to optimize the use of imaging to differentiate benign from malignant causes. Not all masses can be diagnosed with confidence with imaging alone. Because it is not feasible to follow every incidental renal mass, some need to be presumed benign. However, some physicians may be unwilling to accept any diagnostic uncertainty in diagnosis, even though the chance of serious disease is very low. Nevertheless, we believe that the guidelines presented here are practical and medically sound. We emphasize that the guidelines and recommendations included in this review do not necessarily apply to all patients. Each patient's renal mass should be managed individually taking into consideration patient factors and the preferences, capabilities, and expertise of all physicians caring for the patient. As with any set of guidelines aimed to summarize a complicated medical management issue, deviation from the guidelines is inevitable in some patients. With advances in state-of-the art imaging, diagnosis, and treatment of renal masses, it is expected that the guidelines for the management of incidental renal masses will also evolve.

REFERENCES

1. Kissane JM. Congenital malformations. In: Hepinstall RH, editor. Pathology of the kidney. Boston: Little, Brown; 1974. p. 69–119.

2. Tada S, Yamagishi J, Kobayashi H, et al. The incidence of simple renal cysts by computed tomography. Clin Radiol 1983;34:437–9.

3. Jayson M, Sanders H. Increased incidence of serendipitously discovered renal cell carcinoma. Urology 1998;51:203.

4. Konnak JW, Grossman HB. Renal cell carcinoma as an incidental finding. J Urol 1985;134:1094–6.

5. Luciani LG, Cestari R, Tallarigo C. Incidental renal cell carcinoma-age and stage characterization and clinical implications: study of 1092 patients (1982–1997). Urology 2000;56:58–62.

6. Rodriguez-Rubio FI, Diez-Caballero F, Martin-Marquina A, et al. Incidentally detected renal cell carcinoma. Br J Urol 1996;78:29–32.

7. Israel GM, Bosniak MA. How I do it: evaluating renal masses. Radiology 2005;236:441–50.

8. Bae KT, Heiken JP, Siegel CL, et al. Renal cysts: is attenuation artifactually increased on contrast-enhanced CT images? Radiology 2000;216:792–6.

9. Maki DD, Birnbaum BA, Chakraborty DP, et al. Renal cyst pseudoenhancement: beam-hardening effects on CT numbers. Radiology 1999;213:468–72.

10. Birnbaum BA, Hindman N, Lee J, et al. Renal cyst pseudoenhancement: influence of multidetector CT reconstruction algorithm and scanner type in phantom model. Radiology 2007;244:767–75.

11. Birnbaum BA, Hindman N, Lee J, et al. Multi-detector row CT attenuation measurements: assessment of intra- and interscanner variability with an anthropomorphic phantom. Radiology 2007;242:109–19.

12. Hecht EM, Israel GM, Krinsky GA, et al. MR imaging of renal masses: comparison of quantitative enhancement using signal intensity measurements versus qualitative enhancement with image subtraction. Radiology 2004;232:373–8.

13. Ho VB, Allen SF, Hood MN, et al. Renal masses: quantitative assessment of enhancement with dynamic MR imaging. Radiology 2002;224:695–700.

14. Bosniak MA. The current radiological approach to renal cysts. Radiology 1986;158:1–10.

15. Curry NS, Cochran ST, Bissada NK. Cystic renal masses: accurate Bosniak classification requires adequate renal CT. Am J Roentgenol 2000;175:339–42.

16. Siegel CL, McFarland EG, Brink JA, et al. CT of cystic renal masses: analysis of diagnostic performance and interobserver variation. Am J Roentgenol 1997;169:813–8.

17. Koga S, Nishikido M, Inuzuka S, et al. An evaluation of Bosniak's radiological classification of cystic renal masses. BJU Int 2000;86:607–9.

18. Levy P, Helenon O, Merran S, et al. [Cystic tumors of the kidney in adults: radio-histopathologic correlations]. J Radiol 1999;80:121–33 [in French].

19. Bosniak MA. Diagnosis and management of patients with complicated cystic lesions of the kidney. AJR Am J Roentgenol 1997;169:819–21.

20. Israel GM, Bosniak MA. Follow-up CT of moderately complex cystic lesions of the kidney (Bosniak category IIF). AJR Am J Roentgenol 2003;181:627–33.

21. Israel GM, Bosniak MA. Calcification in cystic renal masses: is it important in diagnosis? Radiology 2003;226:47–52.

22. Bosniak MA. The use of the Bosniak classification system for renal cysts and cystic tumors. J Urol 1997;157:1852–3.

23. Hartman DS, Weatherby E III, Laskin WB, et al. Cystic renal cell carcinoma: CT findings simulating a benign hyperdense cyst. AJR Am J Roentgenol 1992;159:1235–7.

24. Jonisch AI, Rubinowitz A, Mutalik P, et al. Can high attenuation renal cysts be differentiated from renal cell carcinoma at unenhanced computed tomography? Radiology 2007;243:445–50.

25. Chung EP, Herts BR, Linnell G, et al. Analysis of changes in attenuation of proven renal cysts on different scanning phases of triphasic MDCT. AJR Am J Roentgenol 2004;182:405–10.

26. Bosniak MA. Difficulties in classifying cystic lesion of the kidney. Urol Radiol 1991;13:91–3.

27. Bosniak MA. Problems in the radiologic diagnosis of renal parenchymal tumors. Urol Clin North Am 1993; 20:217–30.

28. Bosniak MA. The small (less than or equal to 3.0 cm) renal parenchymal tumor: detection, diagnosis, and controversies. Radiology 1991;179:307–17.

29. Silverman SG, Gan YU, Mortele KJ, et al. Renal masses in the adult patient: the role of percutaneous biopsy. Radiology 2006;240:6–22.

30. Bosniak MA, Rofsky NM. Problems in the detection and characterization of small renal masses. Radiology 1996;198:638–41.

31. Rybicki FJ, Shu KM, Cibas ES, et al. Percutaneous biopsy of renal masses: sensitivity and negative predictive value stratified by clinical setting and size of masses. AJR Am J Roentgenol 2003;180:1281–7.

32. Silverman SG, Gan YU, Mortele KJ, et al. Renal mass biopsy in the new millennium: an important diagnostic procedure. In: Ramchandani P, editor. Categorical course in diagnostic radiology: genitourinary radiology. Oak Brook (IL): Radiological Society of North America; 2006. p. 219–36.

33. Silverman SG, Mortele KJ, Tuncali K, et al. Hyperattenuating renal masses: etiologies pathogenesis, and evaluation. Radiographics 2007;27:1131–43.

34. Spaliviero M, Herts BR, Magi-Galluzzi C, et al. Laparoscopic partial nephrectomy for cystic masses. J Urol 2005;174:614–9.

35. Volpe A, Panzarella T, Rendon RA, et al. The natural history of incidentally detected small renal masses. Cancer 2004;100:738–45.

36. Bosniak MA, Birnbaum BA, Krinsky GA, et al. Small renal parenchymal neoplasms: further observations on growth. Radiology 1995;197:589–97.

37. Kassouf W, Aprikian AG, Laplante M, et al. Natural history of renal masses followed expectantly. J Urol 2004;171:111–3.

38. Kunkle DA, Crispen PL, Chen DY, et al. Enhancing renal masses with zero net growth during active surveillance. J Urol 2007;177:849–53 [discussion: 853–4].

39. Wehle MJ, Thiel DD, Petrou SP, et al. Conservative management of incidental contrast-enhancing renal masses as safe alternative to invasive therapy. Urology 2004;64:49–52.

40. Lang EK. Renal cyst puncture studies. Urol Clin North Am 1987;14:91–102.

41. Harisinghani MG, Maher MM, Gervais DA, et al. Incidence of malignancy in complex cystic renal masses (Bosniak category III): should imaging-guided biopsy precede surgery? AJR Am J Roentgenol 2003;180:755–8.

42. Silverman SG, Israel GM, Herts BR, et al. Management of the incidental renal mass. Radiology 2008;249:16–31.

43. Frank I, Blute ML, Cheville JC, et al. Solid renal tumors: an analysis of pathological features related to tumor size. J Urol 2003;170:2217–20.

44. Bracken RB, Chica G, Johnson DE, et al. Secondary renal neoplasms: an autopsy study. South Med J 1979;72:806–7.

45. Mitnick JS, Bosniak MA, Rothberg M, et al. Metastatic neoplasm to the kidney studied by computed tomography and sonography. J Comput Assist Tomogr 1985;9:43–9.

46. Choyke PL, Glenn GM, Walther MM, et al. Hereditary renal cancers. Radiology 2003;226:33–46.

47. Linehan WM, Vasselli J, Srinivasan R, et al. Genetic basis of cancer of the kidney: disease-specific approaches to therapy. Clin Cancer Res 2004;10:6282S–9S.

48. Tickoo SK, Reuter VE, Amin MB, et al. Renal oncocytosis: a morphologic study of fourteen cases. Am J Surg Pathol 1999;23:1094–101.

49. Bosniak MA. Angiomyolipoma (hamartoma) of the kidney: a preoperative diagnosis is possible in virtually every case. Urol Radiol 1981;3:135–42.

50. Bosniak MA, Megibow AJ, Hulnick DH, et al. CT diagnosis of renal angiomyolipoma: the importance of detecting small amounts of fat. AJR Am J Roentgenol 1988;151:497–501.

51. Jinzaki M, Tanimoto A, Narimatsu Y, et al. Angiomyolipoma: imaging findings in lesions with minimal fat. Radiology 1997;205:497–502.

52. Takahashi K, Honda M, Okubo RS, et al. CT pixel mapping in the diagnosis of small angiomyolipomas of the kidneys. J Comput Assist Tomogr 1993;17:98–101.

53. Israel GM, Hindman N, Hecht E, et al. The use of opposed-phase chemical shift MRI in the diagnosis of renal angiomyolipomas. AJR Am J Roentgenol 2005;184:1868–72.

54. Kim JK, Park SY, Shon JH, et al. Angiomyolipoma with minimal fat: differentiation from renal cell carcinoma at biphasic helical CT. Radiology 2004;230:677–84.

55. Fielding JR, Visweswaran A, Silverman SG, et al. CT and ultrasound features of metanephric adenoma in adults with pathologic correlation. J Comput Assist Tomogr 1999;23:441–4.

56. Jinzaki M, Tanimoto A, Mukai M, et al. Double-phase helical CT of small renal parenchymal neoplasms: correlation with pathologic findings and tumor angiogenesis. J Comput Assist Tomogr 2000;24:835–42.

57. Hosokawa Y, Kinouchi T, Sawai Y, et al. Renal angiomyolipoma with minimal fat. Int J Clin Oncol 2002;7:120–3.

58. Amendola MA, Bree RL, Pollack HM, et al. Small renal cell carcinomas: resolving a diagnostic dilemma. Radiology 1988;166:637–41.

59. Shinmoto H, Yuasa Y, Tanimoto A, et al. Small renal cell carcinoma: MRI with pathologic correlation. J Magn Reson Imaging 1998;8:690–4.

60. Yamashita Y, Honda S, Nishiharu T, et al. Detection of pseudocapsule of renal cell carcinoma with MR imaging and CT. AJR Am J Roentgenol 1996;166:1151–5.

61. Yoshimitsu K, Kakihara D, Irie H, et al. Papillary renal carcinoma: diagnostic approach by chemical shift gradient-echo and echo-planar MR imaging. J Magn Reson Imaging 2006;23:339–44.

62. Sussman SK, Glickstein MF, Krzymowski GA. Hypointense renal cell carcinoma: MR imaging with pathologic correlation. Radiology 1990;177:495–7.

63. Liu J, Fanning CV. Can renal oncocytomas be distinguished from renal cell carcinoma on fine-needle aspiration specimens? A study of conventional smears in conjunction with ancillary studies. Cancer 2001;93:390–7.

64. Chow WH, Devesa SS, Warren JL, et al. Rising incidence of renal cell cancer in the United States. JAMA 1999;281:1628–31.

65. Homma Y, Kawabe K, Kitamura T, et al. Increased incidental detection and reduced mortality in renal cancer–recent retrospective analysis at eight institutions. Int J Urol 1995;2:77–80.

66. Chawla SN, Crispen PL, Hanlon AL, et al. The natural history of observed enhancing renal masses: meta-analysis and review of the world literature. J Urol 2006;175:425–31.

67. Siu W, Hafez KS, Johnston WK III, et al. Growth rates of renal cell carcinoma and oncocytoma under surveillance are similar. Urol Oncol 2007;25:115–9.

68. Gill IS, Aron M, Bervais DA, et al. Small renal mass. N Engl J Med 2010;362:624–34.

69. Hsu RM, Chan DY, Siegelman SS. Small renal cell carcinomas: correlation of size with tumor stage, nuclear grade, and histologic subtype. AJR Am J Roentgenol 2004;182:551–7.

70. Birnbaum BA, Bosniak MA, Megibow AJ, et al. Observations on the growth of renal neoplasms. Radiology 1990;176:695–701.

71. Wills JS. Management of small renal neoplasms and angiomyolipoma: a growing problem. Radiology 1995;197:583–6.

72. Francis IR, Choyke P, Bluth E, et al. Indeterminate renal masses. ACR appropriateness criteria, summary of literature review. Reston (VA): American College of Radiology; 2005.

73. Novick AC, Campbell SC, Belldegrun A, et al. Guideline for management of the clinical stage 1 renal mass. J Urol 2009;182(4):1271–9.

Index

Note: Page numbers of article titles are in **boldface** type.

Radiol Clin N Am 49 (2011) 385–389
doi:10.1016/S0033-8389(11)00011-X
0033-8389/11/$ – see front matter © 2011 Elsevier Inc. All rights reserved.

radiologic.theclinics.com

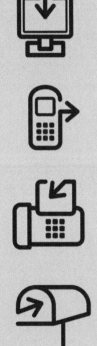

Printed and bound by CPI Group (UK) Ltd, Croydon, CR0 4YY

03/10/2024

01040357-0018